Anatomy for problem solving in sports medicine

The knee

Other books from M&K include

Practical Prescribing for Musculoskeletal Practitioners 2/e
ISBN: 9781905539789

Clinical Examination Skills for Healthcare Professionals
ISBN: 9781905539710

Routine Blood Results Explained 3/e
ISBN: 9781905539888

The ECG Workbook 2/e
ISBN: 9781905539772

Anatomy for problem solving in sports medicine

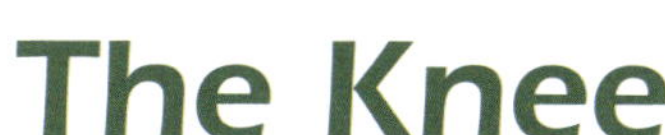

The Knee

Philip Harris
Craig Ranson
Angus Robertson

Title Anatomy for problem solving in sports medicine: The knee
Author **Professor Philip Harris, Dr Craig Ranson and Mr Angus Robertson**

ISBN: 9781905539-89-5

First published 2014

British Library Cataloguing in Publication Data
A catalogue record for this book is available from the British Library

Notice

Clinical practice and medical knowledge constantly evolve. Standard safety precautions must be followed, but, as knowledge is broadened by research, changes in practice, treatment and drug therapy may become necessary or appropriate. Readers must check the most current product information provided by the manufacturer of each drug to be administered and verify the dosages and correct administration, as well as contraindications. It is the responsibility of the practitioner, utilising the experience and knowledge of the patient, to determine dosages and the best treatment for each individual patient. Any brands mentioned in this book are as examples only and are not endorsed by the publisher. Neither the publisher nor the authors assume any liability for any injury and/or damage to persons or property arising from this publication.

To contact M&K Publishing write to:
M&K Update Ltd · The Old Bakery · St. John's Street
Keswick · Cumbria CA12 5AS
Tel: 01768 773030 · Fax: 01768 781099
publishing@mkupdate.co.uk
www.mkupdate.co.uk

Designed and typeset by Mary Blood
Printed in Scotland by Bell & Bain, Glasgow

Contents

Figures

Foreword

When examining patients with sports-related and exercise-related injuries, a thorough knowledge of anatomy has a pivotal role in arriving at a diagnosis and management plan. In this book a professional anatomist, an orthopaedic surgeon and a sports physiotherapist have combined their expertise to present a series of problems related to the sporting knee. The accompanying text provides descriptions and images of the relevant anatomy required to solve each problem. The detail of the content, although clearly and simply presented, goes well beyond the usual descriptive anatomy found in many anatomical textbooks. We hope this book will be a valuable resource for the wide range of health professionals who manage sports-related injuries.

Professor Philip Harris, Dr Craig Ranson and Mr Angus Robertson

The authors would like to thank Dr Peter Mullaney, Consultant Musculoskeletal Radiologist at the Cardiff & Vale NHS Trust for supplying several of the radiological images for the book.

About the authors

Philip Harris

Professor Harris is Emeritus Professor of Anatomy, University of Manchester, a Fellow of the Anatomical Society UK and a past examiner in Anatomy to the Royal Colleges of Surgeons of England, Edinburgh and Glasgow. He has extensive experience of teaching Anatomy to undergraduates and postgraduates over many years. His special interests include applied and living anatomy of the locomotor system and he has taught courses in Sports Medicine and Sports Science. With Dr Ranson, Professor Harris is co-author of the book *Living and Surface Anatomy for Sports Medicine.*

Craig Ranson

Dr Ranson is a Senior Lecturer in Sport and Exercise Medicine at Cardiff Metropolitan University and a Sports Physiotherapist with the Wales Rugby Team. His previous posts include UK Athletics Chief Physiotherapist and National Lead Physiotherapist to the England and Wales Cricket Board. Craig is a consultant to a variety of sporting organisations including the International Cricket Council and the Sports Medicine Department of the University of the West Indies.

Angus Robertson

Mr Robertson is a Consultant in Trauma and Orthopaedics at Cardiff and Vale NHS Trust. He is also managing partner at Cardiff Sports Orthopaedics LLP, an Honorary Senior Lecturer in Sports and Exercise Medicine at Cardiff Metropolitan University and Medical Director at Pontypool RFC. His clinical and research interests include sports injuries, arthroscopy and reconstruction of the knee, shoulder and elbow.

1

Introduction to solving sports injury problems and the role of anatomy

This book presents the structural and functional anatomy of the knee that is particularly relevant to the understanding of sports injuries. When combined with a consideration of the surface and living anatomy of the knee, including special examination tests (Harris & Ranson 2008), this should enable the reader to apply their knowledge when solving problems in a clinical setting.

This book takes a logical approach in order to successfully solve clinical problems. Although each problem is different, practitioners should always follow a similar pattern in arriving at a differential diagnosis. In every case, four main factors need to be kept in mind:

1. The type of sport

2. The clinical history

3. The physical assessment

4. Appropriate investigations

1. The type of sport

Certain structures are more likely to be injured in particular sports. For example, damage to the anterior cruciate ligament is common in sports such as football (soccer) or rugby, where the lower limbs can be subjected to considerable torsional forces.

2. The clinical history

The clinical history must include the mechanism of injury and the presenting symptoms. For instance, sudden torsional loading may damage ligaments or menisci, whereas repetitive minor trauma may result in insertional tendinopathies.

Symptoms of pathology in the knee may include pain, swelling, a feeling of instability or 'giving way', popping, grinding and locking. Pain may be acute, as when a sudden force damages a ligament, or it may be of gradual onset as in progressive damage to articular cartilage (osteoarthritis). Locating the pain is important, and anatomical knowledge can help the practitioner identify the structures that are likely to be involved. For example, pain over the joint line, with precise tenderness over the midpoint on the medial side, suggests damage to the medial collateral ligament or meniscus. Pain and tenderness anteriorly, at the inferior pole of the patella, could indicate patellar tendinopathy.

Generalised swelling of the knee may occur with an effusion, due to excessive fluid (synovial or blood) in the joint, and may be acute or chronic, whereas localised swelling may be as a result of damage to a particular structure such as the medial collateral ligament. Sometimes swelling is associated with inflammation of a bursa, which are particularly common around the knee. A feeling of instability, 'giving way' or 'popping' may result from a ligament strain or rupture so that the articulating surfaces between femur and tibia are no longer optimally stabilised. A grinding sensation in the joint may be caused by damage to the normally ultra-smooth surface of articular cartilage or may result from an unstable meniscal tear. Locking of the joint occurs when it cannot be completely extended. The inability to extend the joint may be caused by a meniscus tear (where a meniscal fragment becomes loose and catches between the articulating surfaces) or it may result from a 'loose body' when a piece of cartilage breaks away and impinges.

3. Physical assessment

Physical assessment includes inspection, manipulation and the use of special techniques and manoeuvres to test specific structures. A knowledge of the functional anatomy of structures is of prime importance in performing and understanding assessment techniques.

4. Appropriate investigations

Appropriate investigations must be selected and interpreted. These include x-rays, Magnetic Resonance Imaging (MRI) and ultrasound scans, as well as direct inspection of the joint using arthroscopic techniques. Images from all these types of investigation cannot be interpreted without a sound knowledge of anatomy.

The use of clinical problems in this book

Clinical problems are presented throughout the book. Each problem provides a clinical history, physical assessment and investigations. Treatment options are given, including the clinical reasoning behind the selection of particular options. Each problem includes a numbered series of questions and answers relating to the findings.

To help the reader, the first problem is presented below as a worked example.

Problem: Worked example

Sport – Football (Soccer)

Clinical history

A 23-year-old accountant sustained a valgus force to his left knee when attempting to tackle an opposing player during a football match two years previously. At the time he experienced immediate pain and could not continue playing. He did not recollect any pre-existing knee symptoms. The knee was moderately swollen the following day, and the swelling persisted for a week. He has not had any treatment to date. The patient continues to complain of pain in the lateral side of his knee. He experiences occasional pain and swelling with activity, and a 'clicking and catching' feeling when weight-bearing and when rotating on the knee.

Q1. What are the possible diagnoses?

Q2. Is the lateral collateral ligament likely to be implicated?

Physical assessment

Examination of the patient revealed normal lower limb alignment, a full range of movement and no instability.

Q3. What special tests or manoeuvres during the examination would be helpful in confirming the diagnosis?

Investigations

The patient's general practitioner has arranged for x-rays to be performed. These have been reported as 'no abnormality detected'.

Q4. What is the next most appropriate investigation and why?

MRI shows the following (see below).

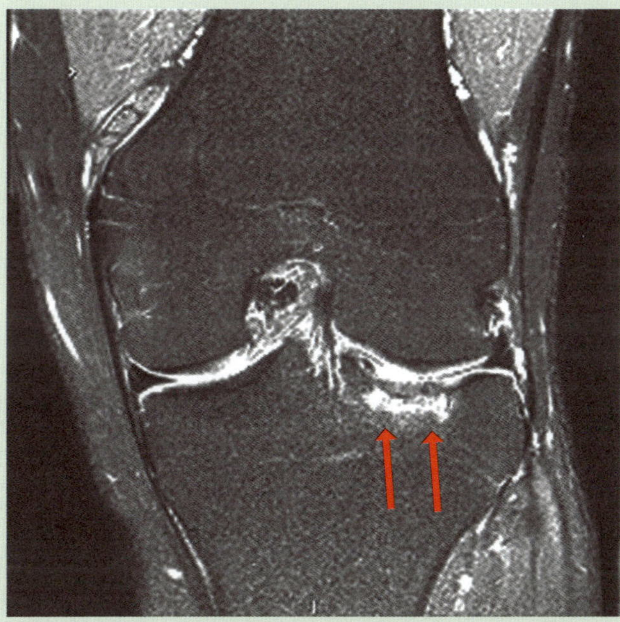

Q5. What diagnosis can be made from the scan?

Treatment

The patient has tried resting the knee and has taken simple analgesics.

Q6. What other treatment options are available?

Worked example: Answers

Diagnosis: Tibial plateau injury.

A1. Lateral meniscal tear

Chondral injury/Osteochondral injury

A2. In a valgus injury, it is more likely that the *medial* collateral ligament is injured, as it is placed under tension. If there is significant depression of the lateral tibial plateau as a result of the injury, the lateral collateral ligament may appear lax, as putting a varus force on the knee results in a return to its normal anatomical position before the ligament starts to be tensioned.

A3. McMurray's test and Apley's grind and distraction tests.

A4. MRI to allow visualisation of the menisci and articular surfaces. An MRI is also useful to assess associated ligamentous structures.

A5. MRI confirms an impaction fracture of the lateral tibial plateau with evidence of subchondral cyst formation.

A6a. Rehabilitation exercises, concentrating on strengthening and improving control of the knee flexors and extensors. Initially the programme might be biased towards open kinetic chain exercises (such as knee extensions and hamstring curls) to allow muscle strengthening without significant axial loading of the damaged joint. If possible, this should progress to include low-impact, high-frequency exercises such as skipping, which might have a positive effect on bone and cartilage synthesis. The later stages should incorporate heavier-load, closed chain exercises such as squats.

A6b. An arthroscopic assessment with debridement or micro-fracture of the chondral lesion may be indicated if the patient's symptoms fail to resolve.

2

Introduction to the anatomy of the knee

In the lower limb the region of the knee marks the transition from the thigh proximally to the leg distally. The bulk of the knee is formed by the knee joint itself, which occupies a crucial position in the lever system of the limb. It is a synovial joint, which functions as a modified hinge with a wide range of movement. The knee facilitates much of the movement required for locomotion, whether walking, running or jumping.

In sport, the knee is one of the most frequently damaged joints. Contributory factors include its vulnerable position in the lever system, its relatively superficial location and the fact that its stability depends considerably on the integrity of its associated ligaments and tendons. It is notably susceptible to torsional (twisting) forces whilst the foot is on the ground, and to forced abduction and adduction forces that commonly occur in the football codes, court sports and martial arts. Excessive forces acting in a sagittal plane may damage the anterior cruciate ligament, an injury commonly seen in alpine skiers and running-based team sports. Sustained or repetitive weight bearing, especially when excessive (as in weight lifting), may result in cumulative damage to articular cartilage. The patellofemoral joint and tendons surrounding the knee are also susceptible to cumulative micro-trauma injury during a wide range of sporting activities including those involving cycling and running.

The knee joint is relatively superficial, from the anterior, medial and lateral aspects, and this facilitates the clinical examination of the joint. The patella anteriorly forms the prominence of the knee, and is also a component of the joint. Posteriorly the joint is much less accessible, being deeply placed in the floor of the popliteal fossa, a crucial space transmitting the major blood vessels and nerve supply from the thigh to the leg and foot. Forming boundaries of the fossa and spanning it from above are the tendons of the hamstring muscles, and from below the proximal parts of the two heads of the gastrocnemius muscle of the calf.

The knee is a synovial joint with two components:

1. Femoro-tibial – between the medial and lateral condyles of the femur and tibia
2. Patello-femoral – between the patella and trochlear groove of the femur.

Note:

The synovial cavities of both components communicate freely (see page 45). The cavity between the respective femoral and tibial condyles is described as having medial and lateral compartments.

Articulating bones

The three articulating bones of the knee joint, femur, tibia and patella are shown in Figure 1. The articular surfaces and relevant features of each bone are illustrated in Figures 2a, 2b and 2c.

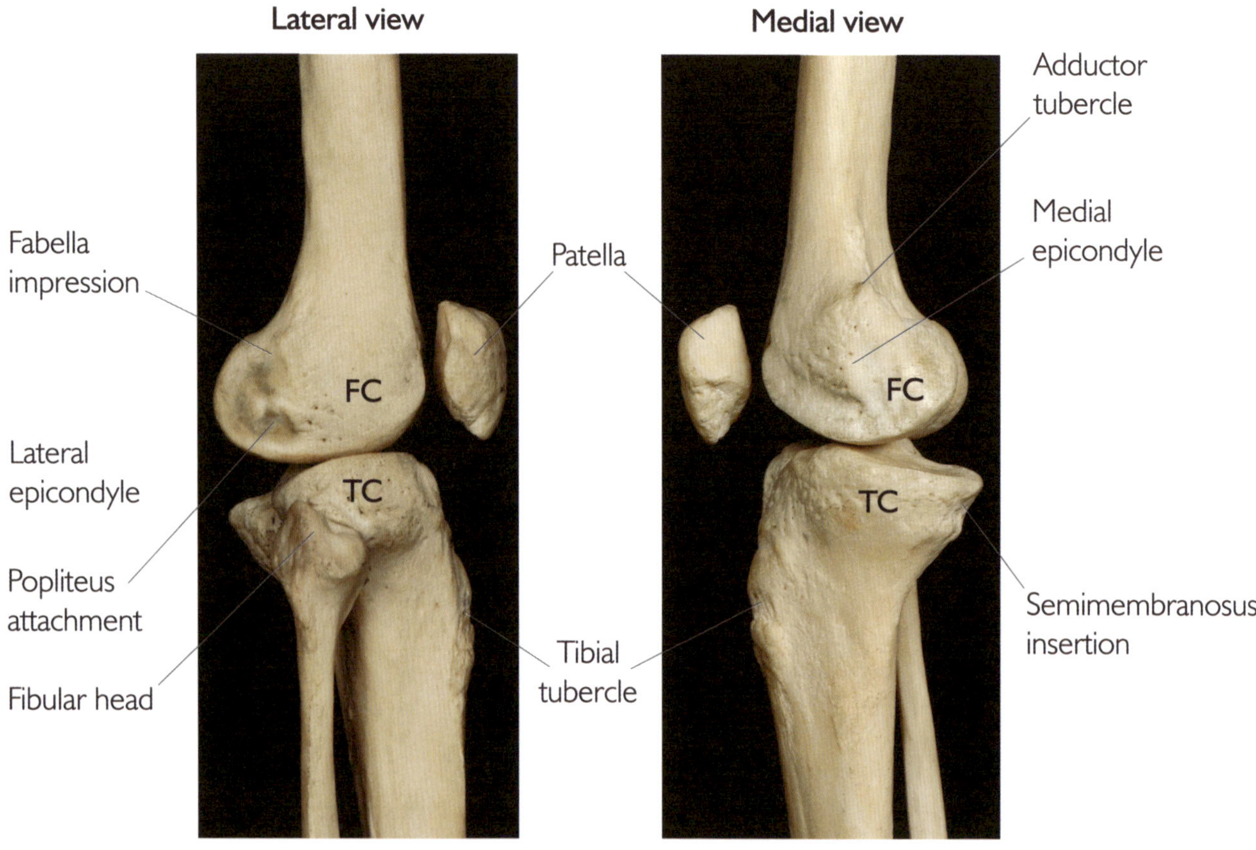

Figure 1. The three articulating bones of the knee joint

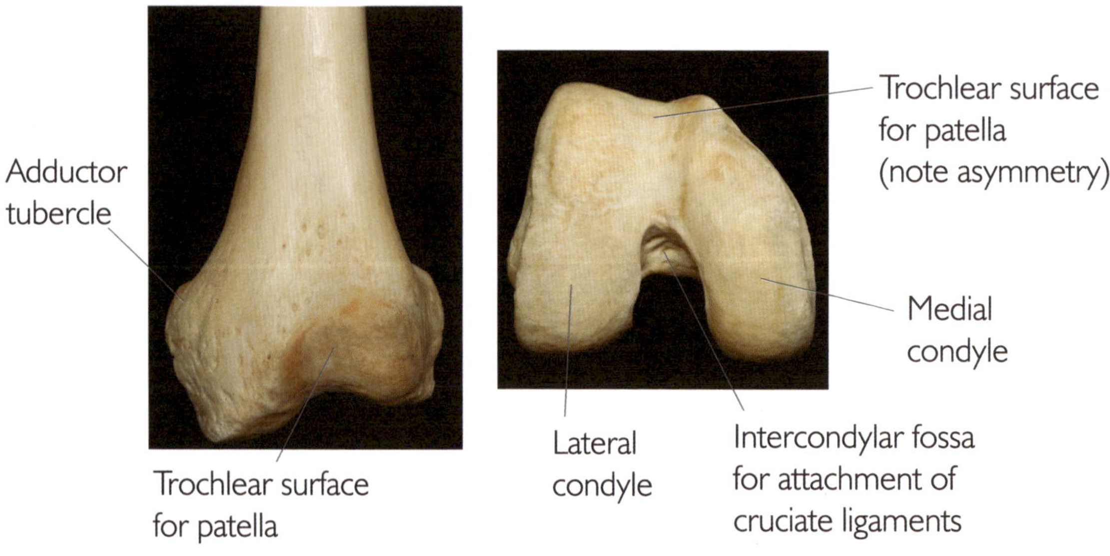

Figure 2a.1: Articulating surfaces of the femur

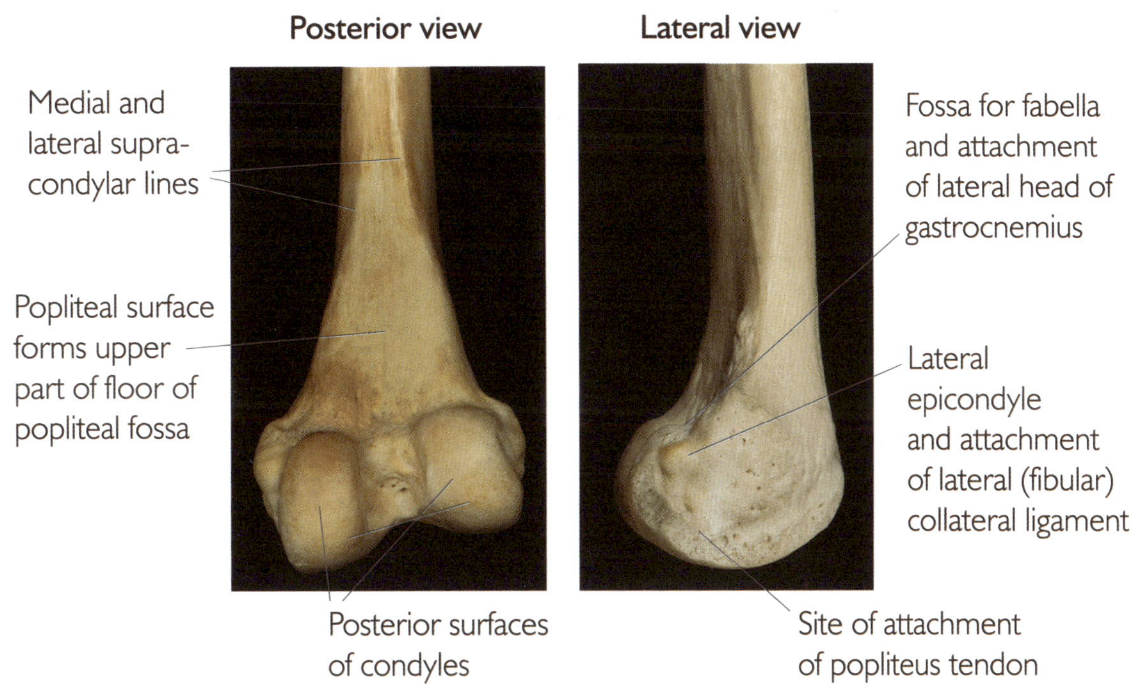

Figure 2a.2: Articulating surfaces of the femur

Features to note on the femur are:

- On the posterior surface of the distal end of the shaft is a broad, flat, triangular area lying between the medial and lateral supracondylar ridges. This forms the upper part of the floor of the popliteal fossa.
- The medial and lateral condyles have extensive articular surfaces since they articulate with two bones, the patella and the tibial condyles. Anteriorly they fuse to form the prominent asymmetrical trochlea, which articulates with the patella. The asymmetry conforms to the similar shape of the patella and relates to the mechanics of the extensor mechanism of the knee (to be considered later, see section 11, page 89). Inferiorly each condyle articulates with the corresponding condyle of the tibia. Here there is also asymmetry, the medial condyle being somewhat larger than the lateral, which is relevant to the mechanics of extension and flexion. Each condyle has a remarkably large articulating surface, the posterior part articulating with the tibial condyles during flexion.
- Between the opposing surfaces of the condyles is a deep intercondylar fossa, which provides anchorage for the cruciate ligaments, the meniscofemoral ligament, and the ligamentum mucosum, which forms the deep extremity of the infra-patellar fat pad.
- On the outer surface of the lateral condyle is a small prominence. This is the lateral epicondyle to which the lateral collateral ligament is attached. Below the epicondyle and therefore within the capsule is a deep groove marking the attachment of the popliteus tendon. Above the epicondyle there is often a round depression marking the location of the fabella, a sesamoid bone in the lateral head of the gastrocnemius muscle.
- On the outer surface of the medial condyle is the prominence of the medial epicondyle and above this at the lower end of the medial supracondylar ridge is the adductor tubercle marking the distal attachment of the adductor magnus.

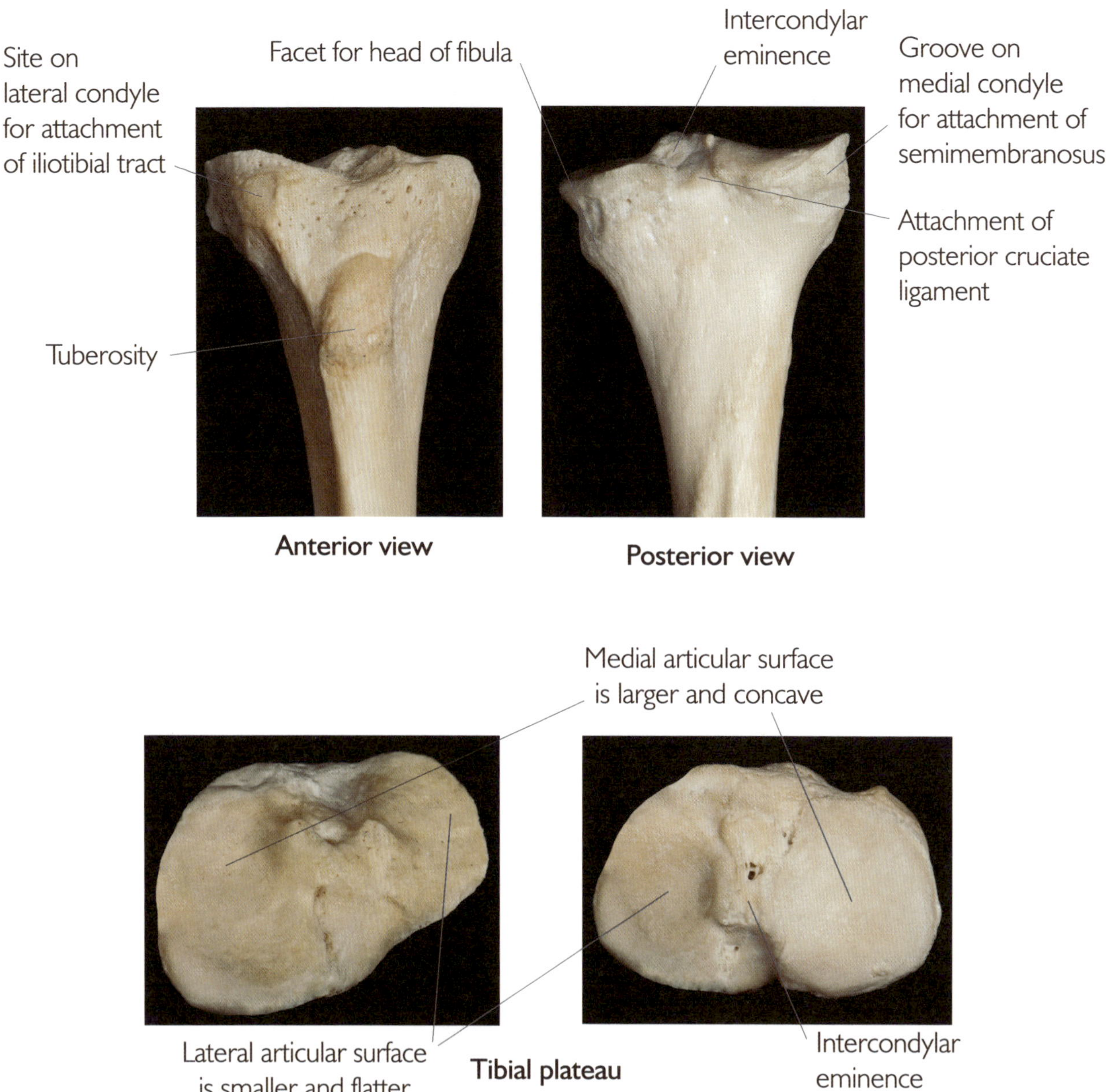

Figure 2b: Articulating surfaces of the tibia

Features to note on the tibia are:

- The articular surfaces on the condyles are different. On the medial side the articular area is larger and slightly concave, whereas on the lateral side it is smaller and flatter. This anatomical difference is important and is relevant to the biomechanics of flexion and extension of the knee.
- The site of attachment of the posterior cruciate ligament behind the articular eminence is large and extends downwards onto the upper part of the shaft beyond the articular margin. This reflects the difference in thickness of the posterior and anterior cruciate ligaments, the posterior being considerably thicker.
- A flat facet, frequently triangular in shape, lies just lateral to the tibial tubercle on the upper part of the lateral condyle, just below the articular margin. This marks the main attachment of the iliotibial band.

Base (upper pole) and attachment of quadriceps tendon
Lateral articular surface is larger
Base
Medial articular surface is smaller
Apex and attachment of patellar tendon
Apex
Anterior surface
Posterior surface

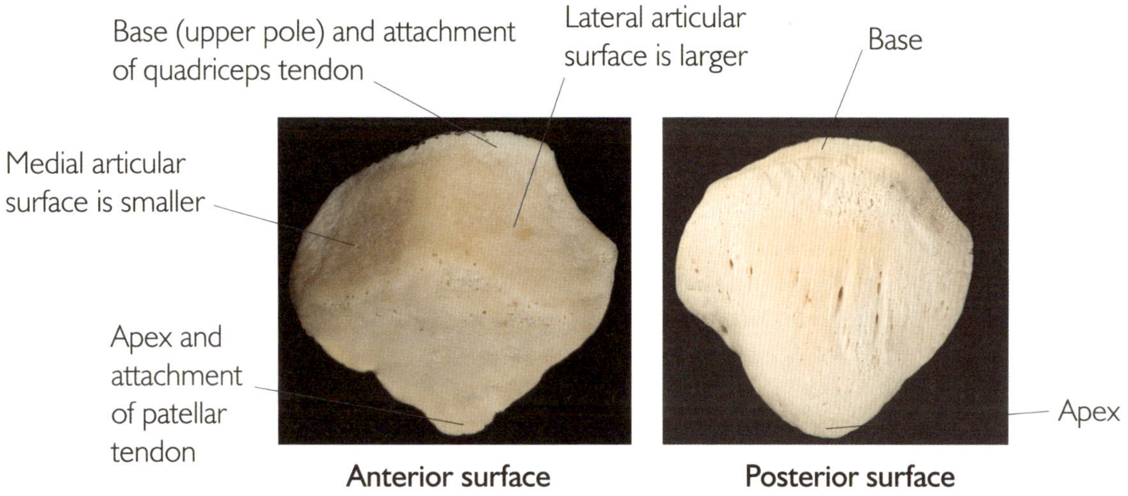

Figure 2c: Patella

Features to note on the patella are:

- The posterior articular surface is asymmetrical, being more extensive on the lateral side.

Articulating surfaces

The articular surfaces of the knee are lined by articular cartilage that macroscopically has a pearly white appearance (see Figures 3a and 3b). It is also known as 'hyaline' cartilage.

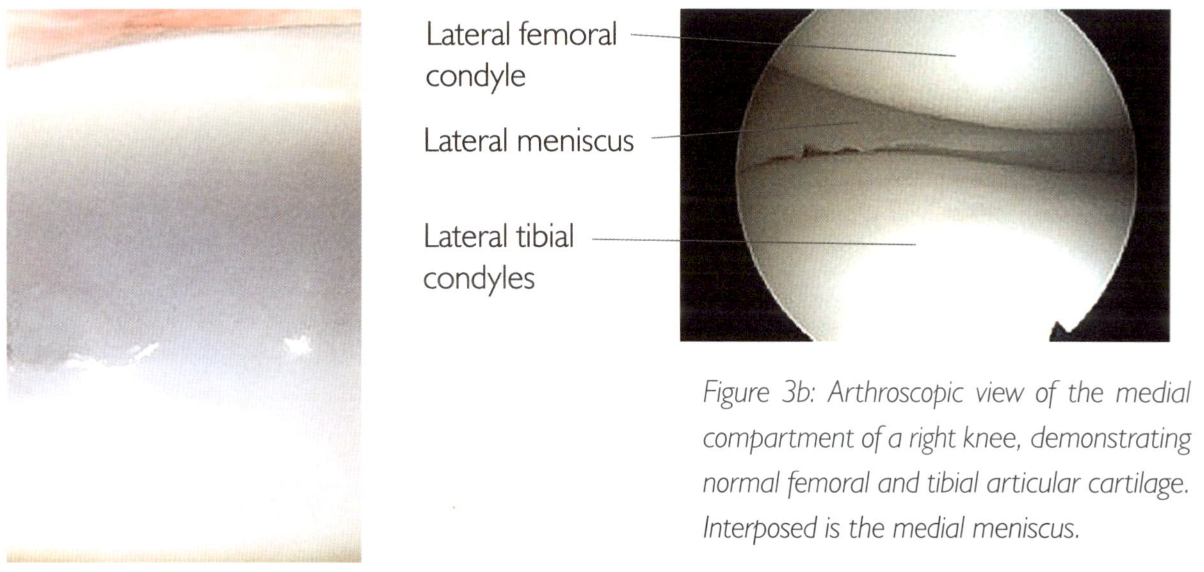

Figure 3b: Arthroscopic view of the medial compartment of a right knee, demonstrating normal femoral and tibial articular cartilage. Interposed is the medial meniscus.

Figure 3a: The in-vivo appearance of articular cartilage

Articular cartilage protects and cushions the underlying bone and is highly compressible, having both permeability and stiffness properties that are related to the water content of the cartilage (about 70%), the amount of collagen (type 2, about 20%) and proteoglycans (about 10%). This composition ensures that relatively large forces are distributed evenly over the articulating surfaces. But the major function of articular cartilage is that, together with the synovial fluid which forms a highly efficient lubricant on its surface, the cartilage ensures almost frictionless movement (Eckstein et al. 2006). The coefficient of friction is extremely low (0.001) and in fact is less than one-third of the coefficient of friction of an ice-to-ice interface!

Articular cartilage is a highly organised, layered structure (see Figures 4a and 4b), which is reflected in its functions. The collagen fibres in the matrix are produced and maintained by the chondrocytes. These are arranged in three layers, each with a specific orientation in respect to the surface. Fibres in the outer layer, next to the joint cavity, are tangential and lie round the circumference. These outer fibres are adapted to shearing forces, as in gliding movements. Those in the middle layer are transitional, lying obliquely and adapted to both shearing and compression forces. Fibres in the deepest layer are radially orientated, lying vertical in respect to the surface, and adapted to compressive force as in weight bearing. Deep to this layer is calcified cartilage and bone.

Unfortunately, articular cartilage injuries have a low healing potential (Perera et al. 2012).

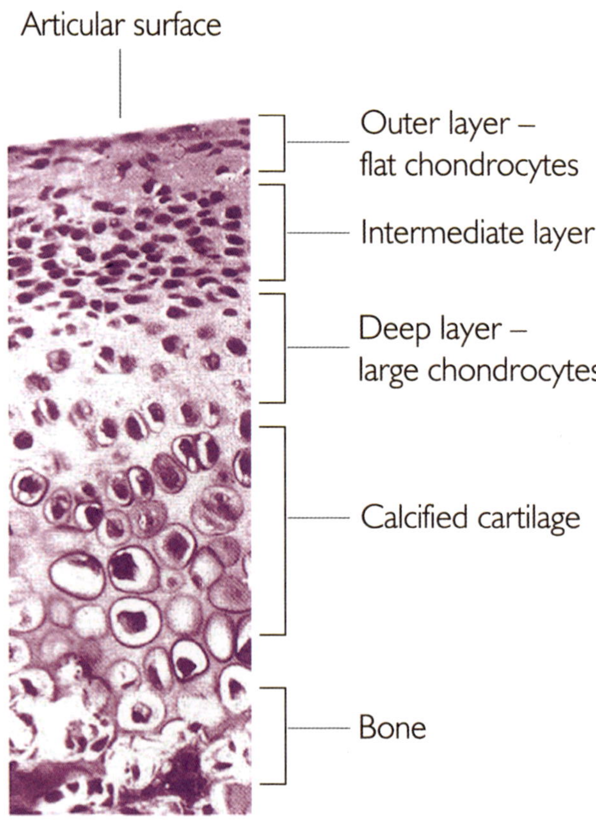

Figure 4a: Histological structure of articular cartilage

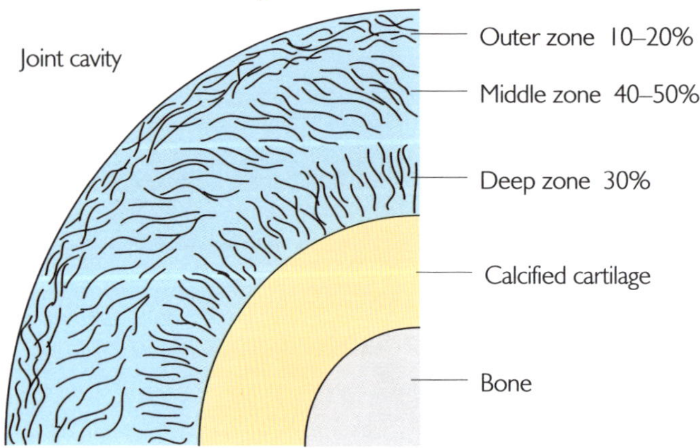

Figure 4b: The orientation of collagen fibres in articular cartilage

Injury to articular cartilage in the knee can vary from small patches of softening or fraying to unstable or loose flaps or even patches of bare bone, where the cartilage has worn away. This can occur through many different mechanisms, including blunt direct or indirect trauma causing anything from minor bruising of the cartilage to major damage such as detachment of a fragment of bone and overlying cartilage – an osteochondral injury (see Figures 5a and 5b). More severe chondral damage can occur in association with dislocation of the patella or ligament injuries such as rupture of the anterior cruciate ligament. This can happen either as a result of direct contusion between the articular surfaces at the time of injury or due to excessive movement between articular surfaces resulting from loss of the normal ligamentous constraints. The cartilage may also be damaged by more chronic conditions such as osteoarthritis. Disruption of articular cartilage structure and function can result in various symptoms, including pain and joint swelling. The joint may click and feel unstable or 'give way'. Where there is more extensive damage, the knee may become increasingly stiff. If osteochondral fragments detach, they can become loose bodies within the joint. These can impinge between articular surfaces and cause 'locking' in the joint.

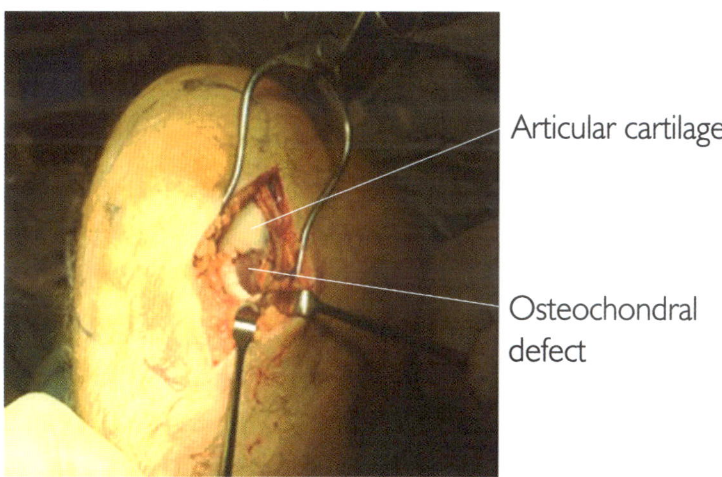

Figure 5a: Operative photograph of a left knee following lateral patellar dislocation, resulting in an osteochondral injury to the lateral femoral condyle

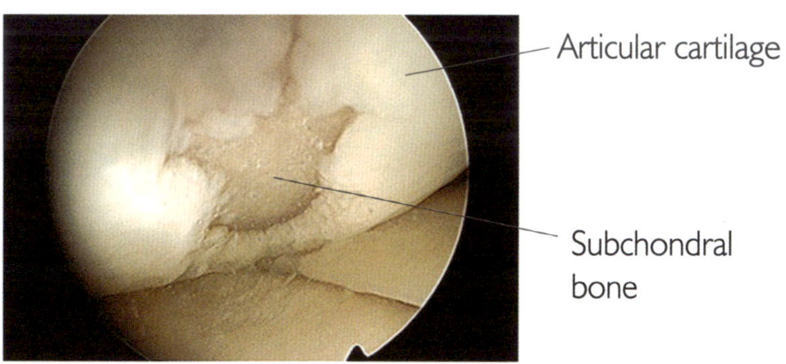

Figure 5b: Arthroscopic view of a full thickness femoral condyle articular cartilage defect

Problem 1

Sport – Motocross

Clinical history

Two months ago, a 34-year-old motocross rider landed heavily from a jump, having had to control the bike by putting his right foot on the ground and thus injuring his right knee. Although the immediate pain and large swelling he experienced have settled, he describes recurrent swelling in the knee when he does any hard riding, running or jumping. There is no 'giving way' or feeling of instability in the knee.

Q1. What symptoms and signs might make you suspect a chondral or osteochondral injury?

Q2. What is the main differential diagnosis?

Examination

Examination reveals a small effusion in the knee. Meniscal provocation and ligament laxity tests are negative.

Q3. What other clinical features might be present on examination of the patient?

Investigations

The man tells you that he is keen to resolve the issue, as he is hoping to become a professional motocross rider shortly.

Q4. What would be the best investigations for this problem and why?

Q5. What does the area indicated by the white arrow in Figure P1.1 demonstrate?

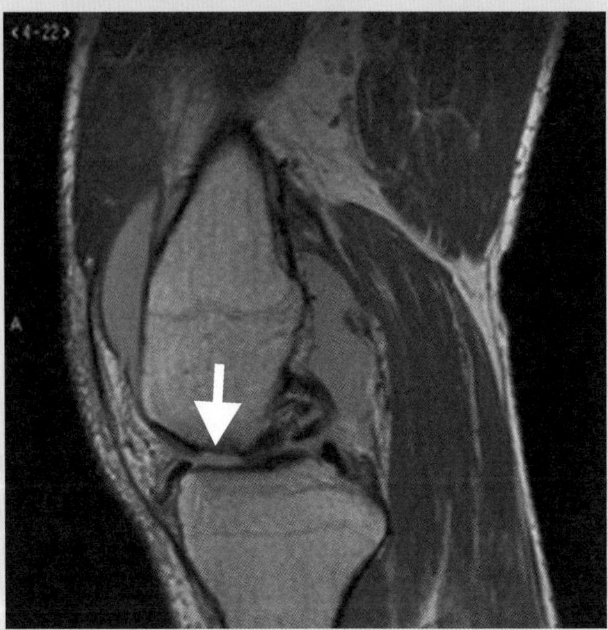

Figure P1.1: Sagittal knee MRI

Treatment

Q6. What treatment options are available?

Answers

Diagnosis: Chondral/Osteochondral injuries

A1. a. Recurrent single joint effusions.

b. Mechanical symptoms ('locking'/'catching').

c. The sensation and/or observation of a 'loose body' within the knee.

A2. One or more meniscal tears.

A3. Joint-line and/or adjacent bony tenderness.

A4. a. X-ray may show compression fractures and ossified loose bodies (beware the normal fabella!).

b. An MRI scan is most useful, as it will detect ossified and non-ossified loose bodies and can often determine their site of origin.

A5. An MRI demonstrating loss of the femoral chondral surface (see Figure P1.1). This correlates with the arthroscopic findings of a full thickness 2 x 2 cm articular cartilage lesion (see Figure P1.2)

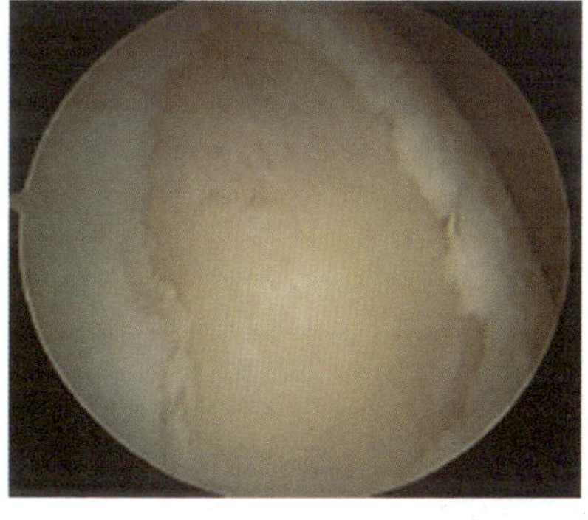

Figure P1.2: Arthroscopic image of a full thickness 2 x 2cm articular cartilage lesion

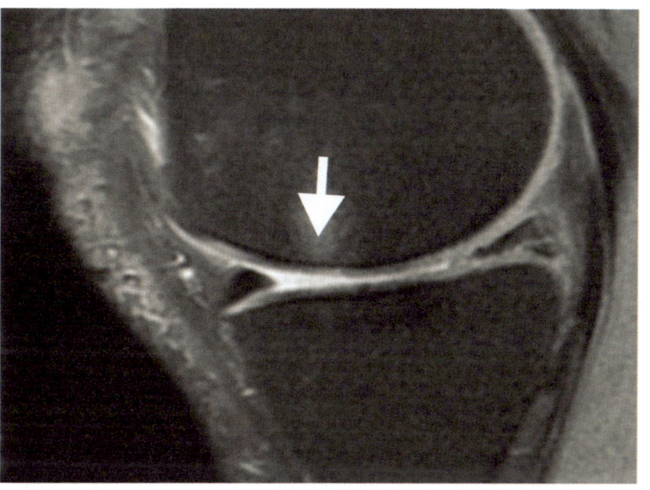

Figure P1.3: Healing area (white arrow) of articular cartilage defect seen in Figures P1.1 and P1.2

A6. a. Removal and treatment of the donor site with microfracture or chondrocyte implantation. In this case, microfracture was performed using a supportive polymer fleece impregnated with hyaluronic acid. Six months postoperatively the patient demonstrated good MRI evidence of infill of the defect (see Figure P1.3). He also had full resolution of symptoms with a return to normal function.

b. In larger fragments reattachment using bioabsorbable implants may be possible.

The normal smooth surface of articular cartilage imparts the clean contours of the articular surfaces of the femur, tibia and patella as seen on x-rays of the knee (see Figures 6a, 6b and 6c).

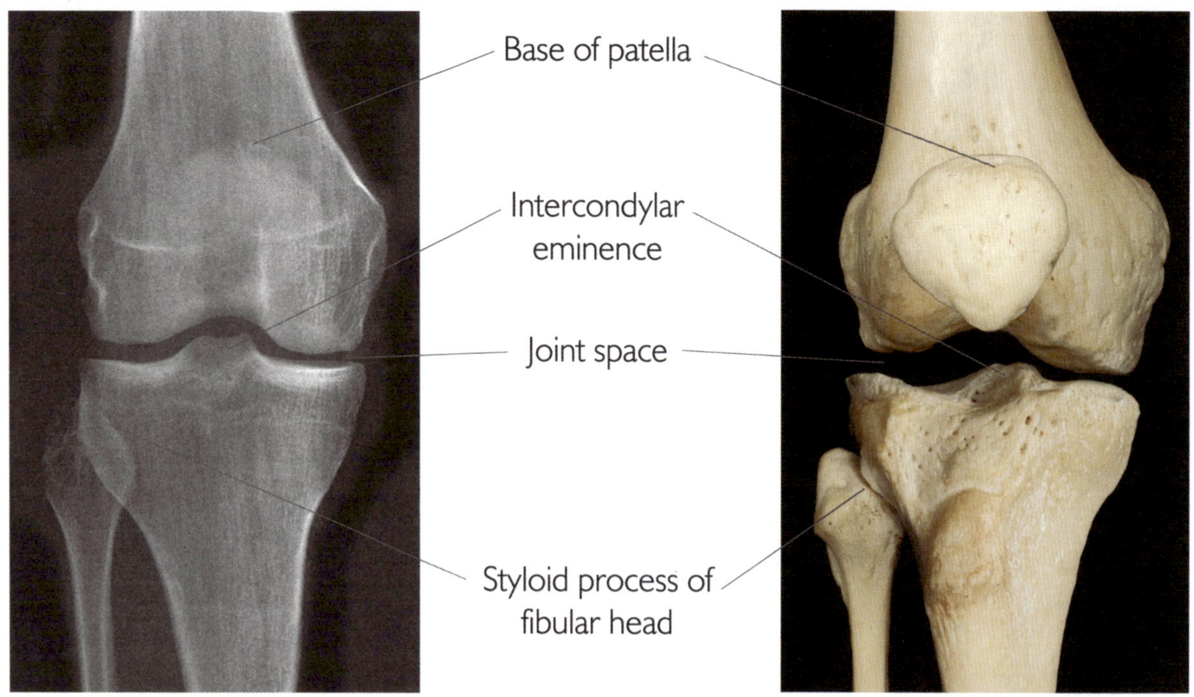

Figure 6a: Antero-posterior weight-bearing radiograph and articulated skeleton of a normal right knee

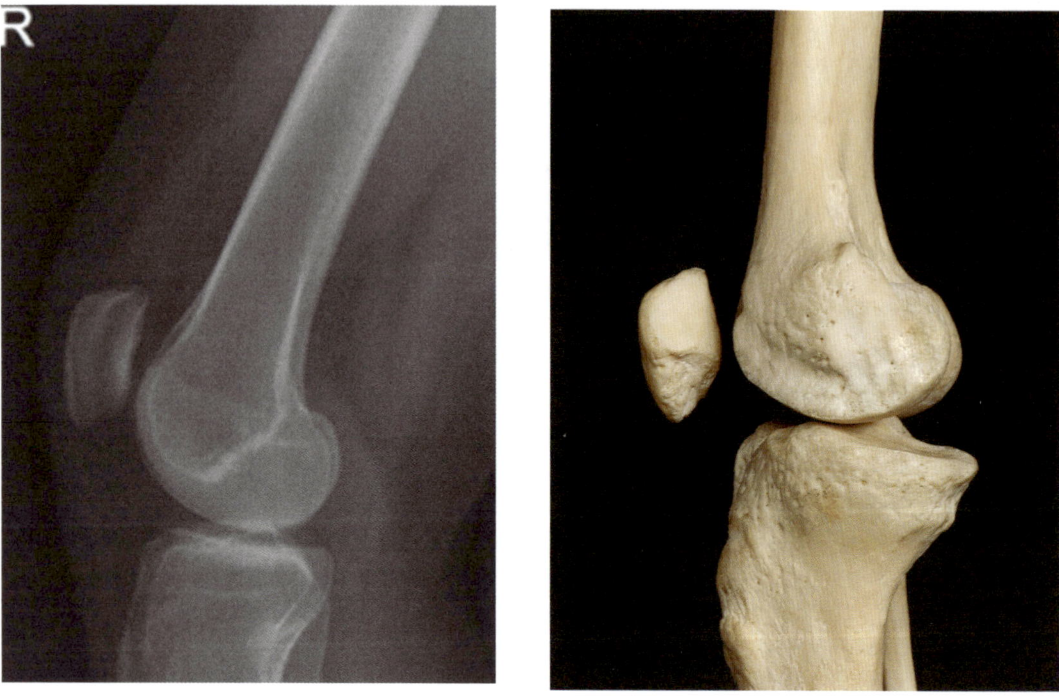

Figure 6b: Lateral weight-bearing radiograph and articulated skeleton of a normal right knee

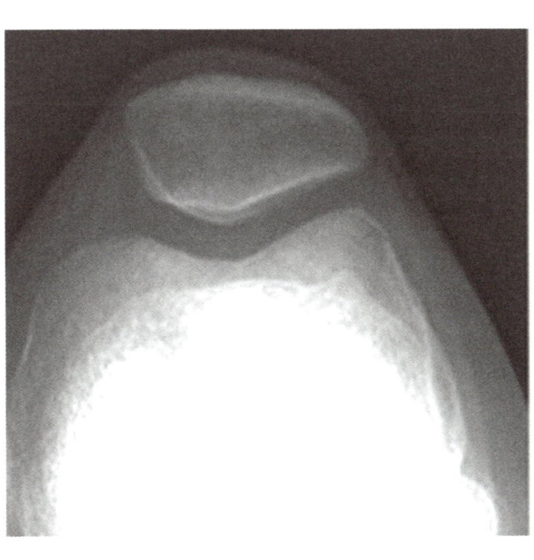

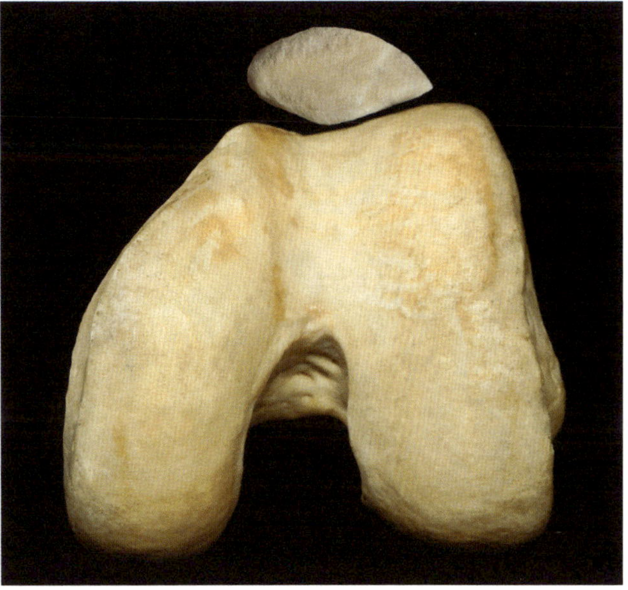

Figure 6c: 'Skyline' radiograph and articulated skeleton of a normal left knee

Problem 2

Sport – cricket

Clinical history

A 16-year-old boy presents with a 12-month history of antero-medial knee pain. He is an active sportsman who regularly plays cricket and rugby. The pain is increased by activity and his parents tell you that he often limps at the end of a sport session. He does not describe any instability or locking but says that his knee 'clicks'.

Examination

Physical examination reveals normal lower limb alignment. There is a small effusion in the knee and pain over the antero-medial portion of the knee to palpation. Meniscal provocation tests are negative and there is no evidence of instability.

Q1. What are the differential diagnoses?

Investigations

Q2. What would be the most helpful investigations and why?

Treatment

Q3. What is the diagnosis (see Figure P2.1, page 16, white arrow) and what is the cause of this condition?

Q4. What is the most appropriate initial treatment?

Q5. A further MRI is performed nine months later (see Figure P2.2, page 16). What does this demonstrate?

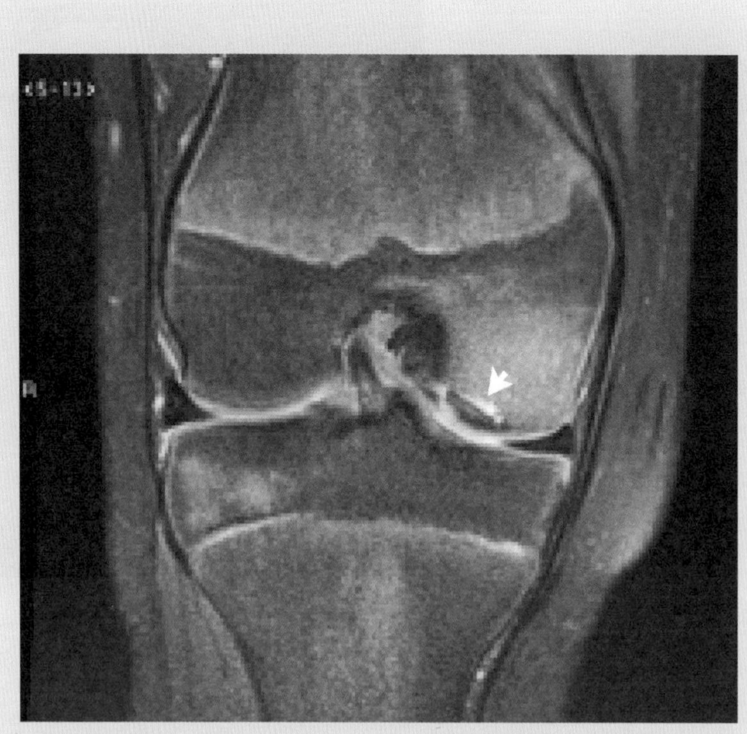

Figure P2.1: Coronal knee MRI

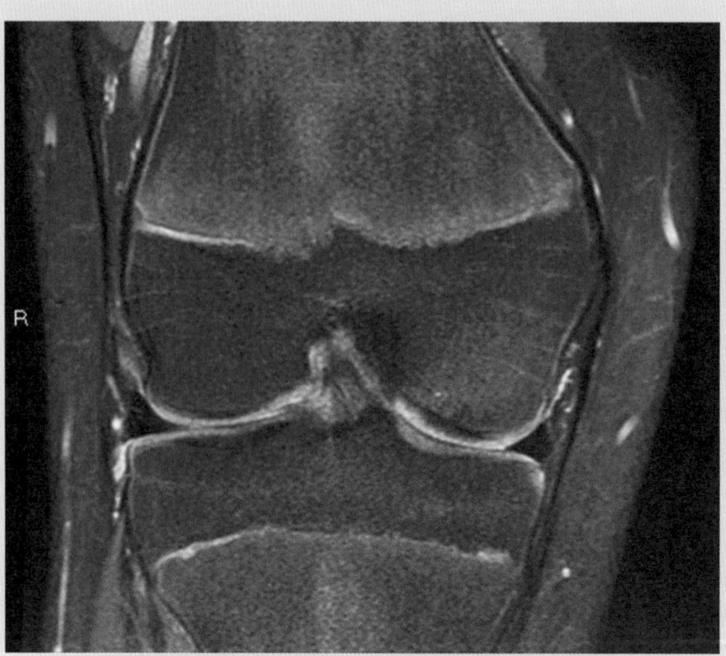

Figure P2.2: Coronal knee MRI

Problem 2: Answers

Diagnosis: Osteochondritis dissecans

A1. a. Medial meniscal pathology.

b. Fat pad impingement.

c. Osteochondritis dissecans (Figure P2.2).

A2. a. Plain x-ray to rule out calcified loose bodies and established osteochondritis dissecans.

b. MRI to confirm the diagnosis.

A3. Osteochondritis dissecans. This is an acquired condition affecting subchondral bone. Initially there is softening of the overlying articular cartilage. This can progress to early articular cartilage separation, partial detachment of an articular lesion, and eventually osteochondral separation with loose bodies. It is a relatively common cause of knee pain and dysfunction in children and adolescents. The aetiology of osteochondritis dissecans is unknown; however, repetitive micro-trauma is often implicated. Osteochondritis dissecans of the knee is subcategorised into a juvenile form and an adult form.

A4. Monitoring, with subsequent radiographic assessment. In juvenile osteochondritis dissecans, more than 50% of cases show healing within six to 18 months with non-operative treatment. Adult osteochondritis dissecans and juvenile osteochondritis dissecans lesions that do not heal have the potential for later sequelae, including osteoarthritis.

A5. Resolution of the lesion.

3

Anterior structures

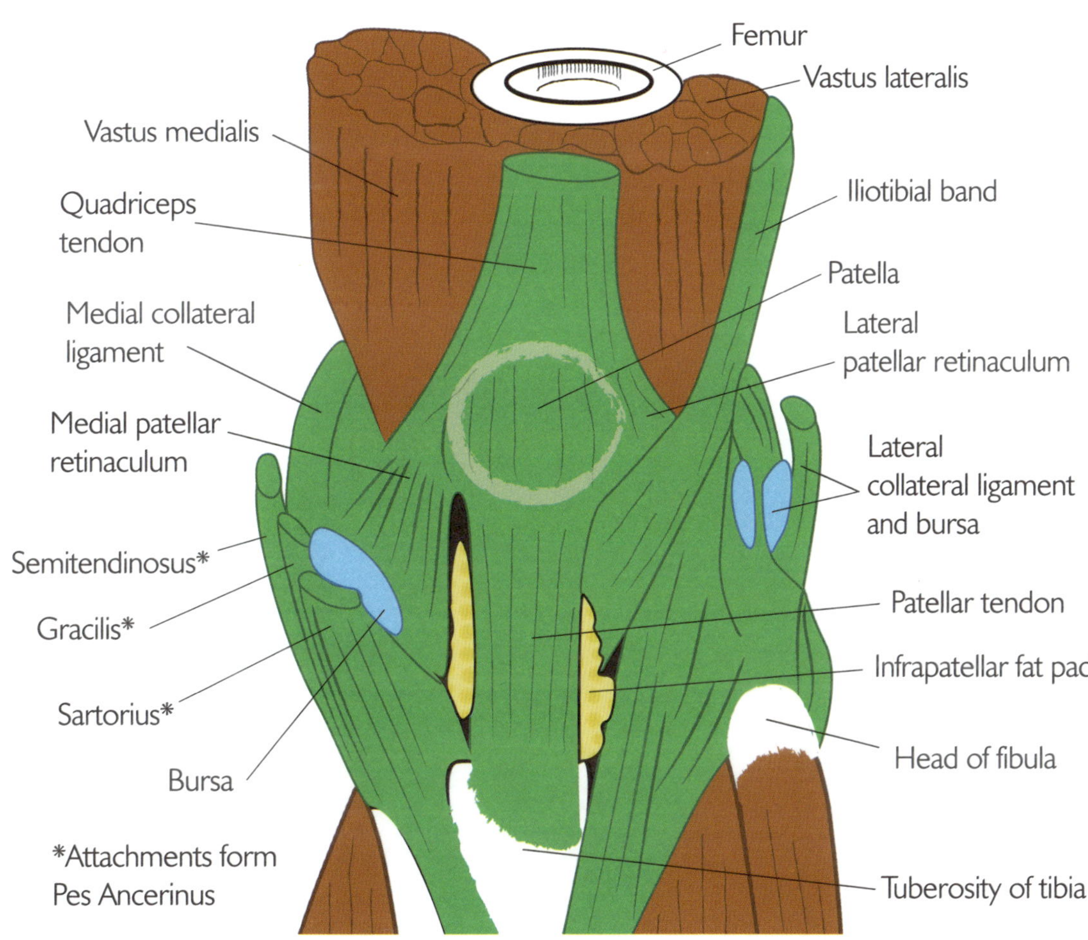

Figure 7: Anterior knee external features: muscles, tendons and associated bursae, ligaments

Several of these structures may be involved in pathology related to participation in sport. Disorders of the patella itself will be considered in Section 11, where its role in relation to the knee joint is discussed. Pain at the inferior pole of the patella is often associated with patellar tendinopathy. It is particularly prevalent amongst athletes in jumping sports such as volleyball, basketball and the jumping field events in athletics. A continuum of pathological change within the patellar tendon is described by Cook & Purdam (2008), ranging from acute reversible tendon swelling that occurs in response to an acute overloading of the tendon to more irreversible degenerative tendon disease characterised by tendinosis and neo-vascularisation (see Figures 8 and 9a, 9b and 9c), thought to be due to the accumulative effects of chronic microtrauma (Cook & Purdam 2008).

Other causes of superficial anterior knee pain in the exercising population include prepatellar bursitis (see Figures 25, 26 and 27, pages 48, 49), which may occur due to recurrent compression in sports where kneeling is frequent, or acutely due to a blow or a fall onto the patella.

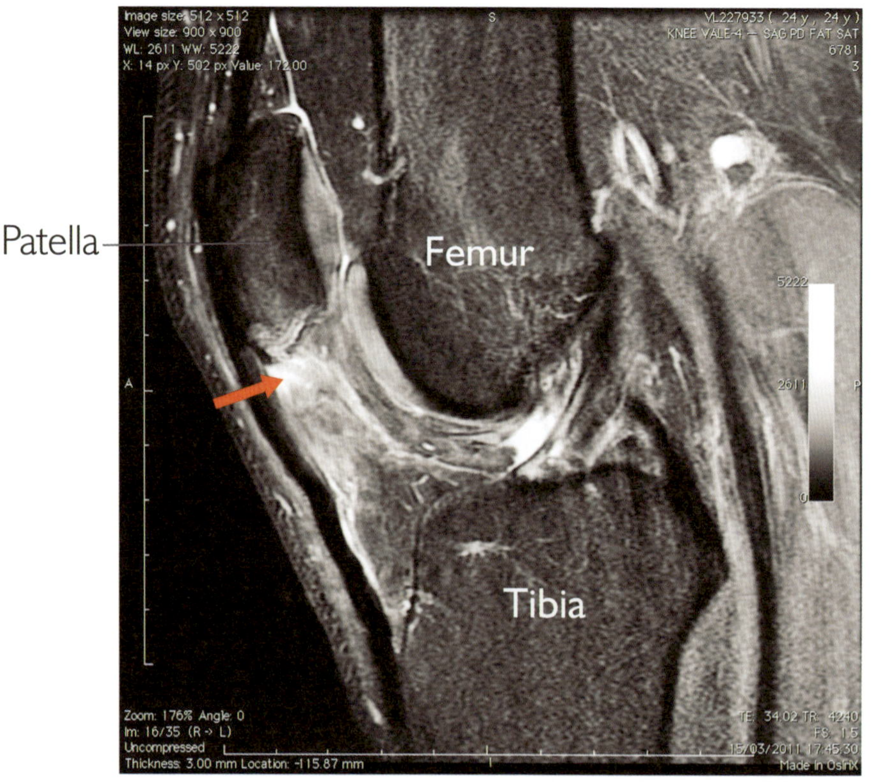

Figure 8: Sagittal magnetic resonance image of patellar tendinopathy.
Note thickened tendon with high-signal intensity indicating oedema deep to the tendon (red arrow).

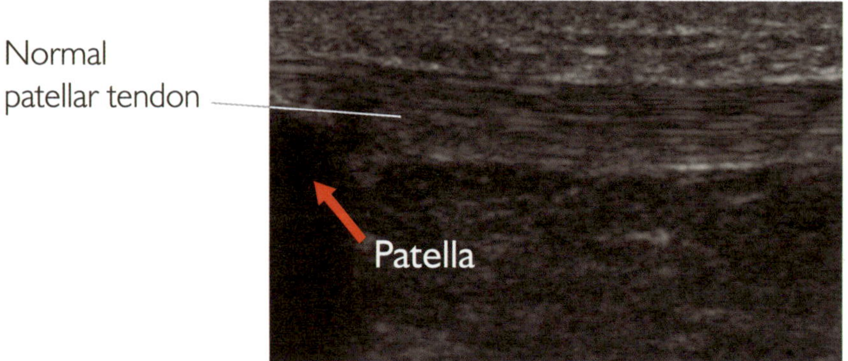

Figure 9a: Sagittal ultrasound image of a normal patellar tendon

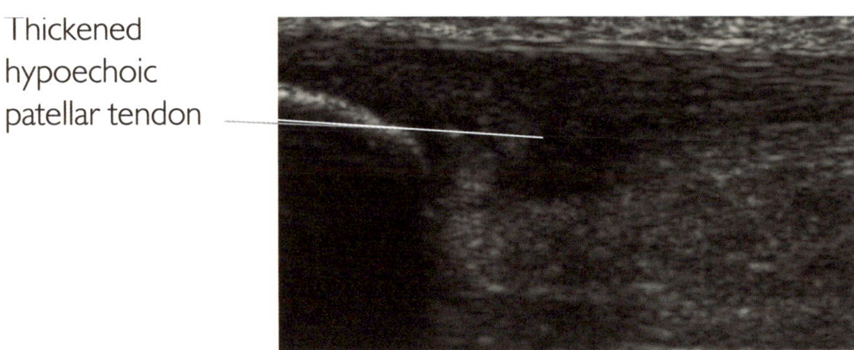

Figure 9b: Sagittal ultrasound image of patellar tendinopathy. Note calcified and thickened tendon with hypoechoic area in the deep tendon indicating tendinosis.

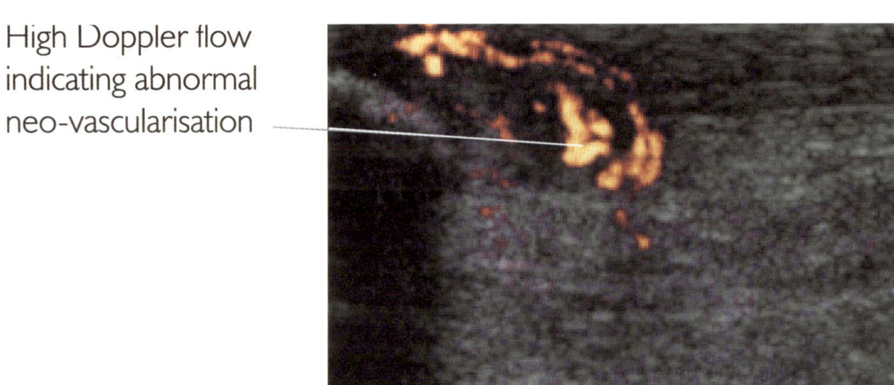

Figure 9c: Sagittal Doppler ultrasound image of patellar tendinopathy. Note florid neo-vascularisation of the tendon emanating from the fat pad below.

Activity-related pain, tenderness and swelling over the inferior pole of the patella or tibial tuberosity in adolescents may be due to proximal (Sinding-Larsen-Johansson disease) or distal (Osgood-Schlatter's disease) apophysitis of the patellar tendon (see Figures 10a, 10b and 11, pages 23,25).

Problem 3

Sport – Running

Clinical history

A 35-year-old male office worker who is a keen recreational runner complains of right anterior knee pain in the infra-patellar region. He describes a gradual onset of pain over a period of six months and does not recall any particular injury. The pain is becoming increasingly severe and longer lasting and is preventing him from training. He has tried resting the knee for a number of weeks without any resolution. He does not have a prior history of knee problems.

Q1. Which structures in the knee could be responsible for these symptoms?

Q2. Which remote regional pathologies need to be considered in this case?

Physical assessment

Examination reveals midline tenderness of the proximal patellar tendon with some localised swelling.

Q3. What are the most likely diagnoses?

Investigations

A colleague has arranged for a plain radiograph, which was unremarkable, and the patient has had a Doppler ultrasound scan, which was reported as showing typical features of 'patellar tendinopathy' (see Figures 9b and 9c, page 21).

Q4. What might these features be and why might they be present?

Q5. What other type of investigation might be useful ?

Treatment

Q6. What treatment options are available?

Q7. What is the likely period of recovery?

Problem 3: Answers

Diagnosis: Patellar tendinopathy

A1. a. Patellofemoral joint (trochlea or retro-patellar joint surfaces).
b. Medial or lateral patellar retinaculum.
c. Patellar tendon.
d. Inferior pole of the patella, or tibial tuberosity entheses of the patellar tendon (Osgood-Schlatter's or Sinding-Larsen-Johansson disease).
e. Anterior knee joint 'Hoffa's' fat pad.
f. Prepatellar bursa.
g. Infrapatellar bursa.
h. Pes-anserina bursa.

A2. a. Referred pain from the hip.
b. Referred pain from the lumbar spine (L3).

A3. a. Patellar tendinopathy.
b. Infrapatellar bursitis.
c. Patellofemoral joint derangement.

A4. a. Thickening of the tendon due to increased water and ground substance content.
b. Hypo-echoicity of the deep one-third of the proximal tendon due to tendinosis.
c. Neo-vascular infiltration of the deep third of the tendon as part of a 'failed or failing' healing response.

A5. An MRI scan can also be helpful in confirming the diagnosis (see Figure 8, page 20) and ruling out additional pathology such as infrapatellar bursitis or patellofemoral joint derangement.

A6. a. Modification of training programme (intensity and duration). Exercise-based tendon rehabilitation programme.

b. Injection therapy, e.g. high volume injection posterior to the patellar tendon.

c. Correction of biomechanical contributors via e.g. exercise rehabilitation or orthothes.

d. Extra-corporeal shock wave therapy.

e. Surgery, e.g. tendon decompression/tenotomy.

A7. Even with optimal treatment, recovery can take a long time. The patient must adhere to their treatment programme and most should begin to experience some improvement in symptoms after a six-week period.

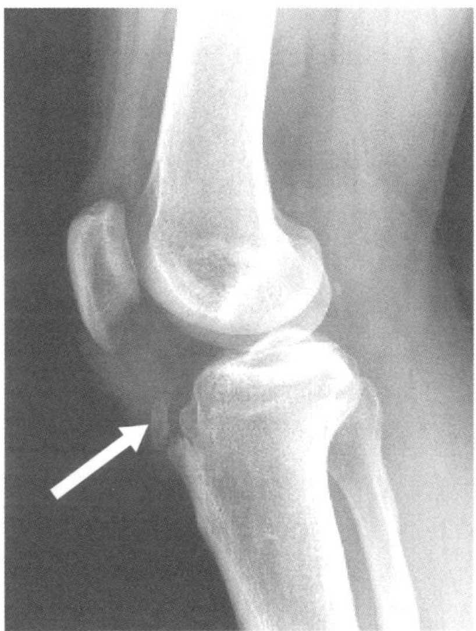

Figure 10a: Lateral radiograph of knee demonstrating Osgood-Schlatter's disease

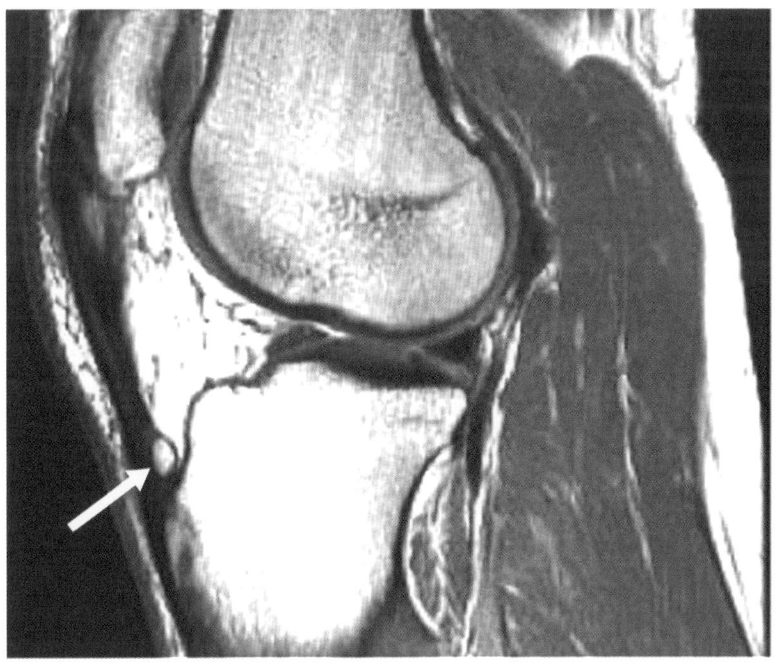

Figure 10b: MRI demonstrating Osgood-Schlatter's disease (white arrow)

Problem 4

Sport – Football (Soccer)

Clinical history

A 23-year-old man presents with pain in the anterior aspect of his knee. He is a keen football player and reports having had 'knee problems' since he was young. He has had tender 'lumps' on the front of his knees since his mid-teens.

Q1. What additional information could the patient usefully provide?

Examination

Clinical examination reveals a bony prominence of the tibial tubercle (see Figure 11).

Q2. What is the most likely diagnosis?

Investigations

In order to support the clinical diagnosis, an x-ray is requested (see Figure 10b).

Q3. What does this demonstrate?

Treatment

The patient is keen to continue to play football and is worried about the lumps. He would like to know more about his condition.

Q4. What is the aetiology of his problem?

Q5. What treatment options are available?

Problem 4: Answers

Diagnosis: Osgood-Schlatter's disease

A1. a. Is there a history of trauma?

b. Are the lumps painful? In particular, is there pain at night?

c. Are they constant or intermittent in nature?

d. What functional effect are the lumps having?

A2. Osgood Schlatter's disease.

A3. Loose ossicle in association with the insertion of the patellar tendon, confirming the diagnosis of Osgood-Schlatter's disease. An MRI can also be useful in confirming the diagnosis and looking for associated pathology (see Figure 10a, page 23). Pes anserine bursitis (see Figure P4.1, curved arrows) can cause swelling medial to the tubercle but can be distinguished by its anatomical location and the 'soft' nature of the swelling.

A4. The condition is caused by stress on the patellar tendon's insertion into the immature tibial tuberosity. This can cause multiple sub-acute avulsion fractures along with inflammation of the tendon, leading to excess bone growth in the tuberosity, which can produce a visible lump that can be painful when hit. Activities such as kneeling may irritate the tendon. The syndrome may develop without trauma or other apparent cause. However, some studies report that up to 50% of patients relate a history of precipitating trauma.

A5. The condition is usually self-limiting. Initial treatment in the acute phase may include rest, ice, compression and elevation (RICE), modification of activities and simple oral analgesics. Bracing may be used to unload the tibial tubercle. Once the symptoms have resolved, a gradual return to sporting activity may be instituted. Predisposing factors should be addressed. Surgery may be required in some cases to excise bony or cartilaginous 'ossicles'.

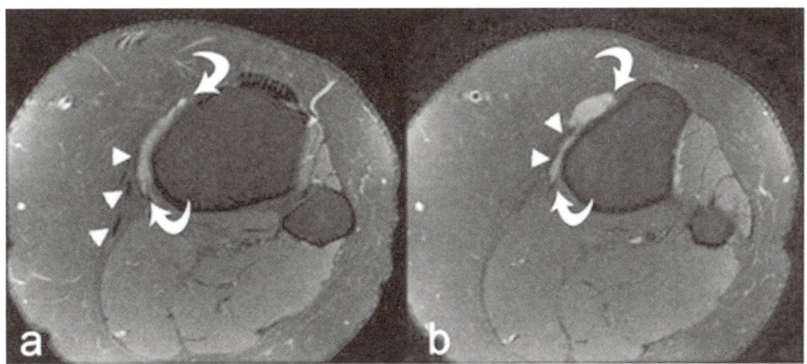

Figure P4.1:
Axial MRI through the proximal tibia, showing swelling of the pes anserine bursa (curved arrows)

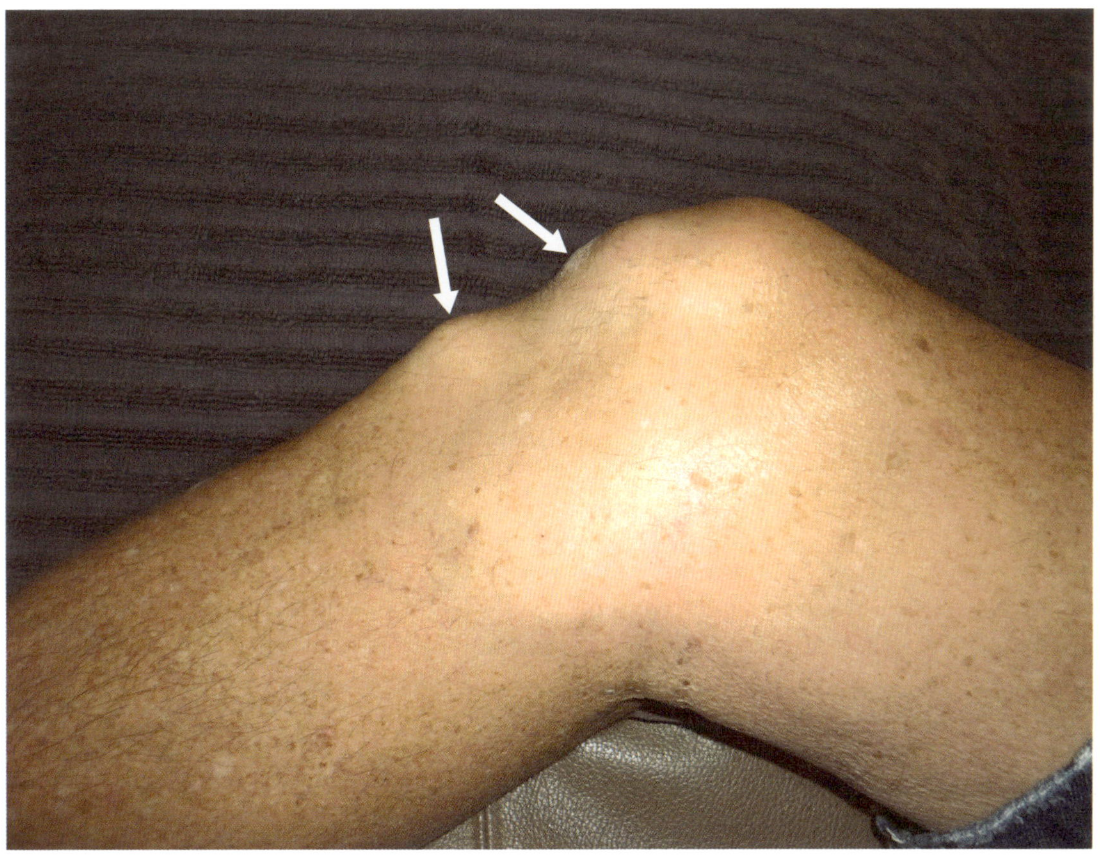

Figure 11: Bony prominences associated with long standing apophysitis of the patellar tendon attachments at the inferior pole of the patella (Sinding-Larsen-Johansson disease – see upper arrow) and tibial tuberosity (Osgood-Schlatter's disease – see lower arrow).

Problem 5

Sport – Cycling

Clinical history

An endurance road cyclist developed lateral knee pain six months ago after slightly raising his seat height before embarking on a two-week alpine tour, covering approximately 150 kilometres per day. He does not recollect any particular trauma but found that each day his pain increased as the day progressed. Eventually the pain began to persist after activity.

Examination

Clinical examination revealed good muscle bulk around the knee, with no evidence of an effusion. There was a small amount of localised swelling over the lateral femoral condyle with associated tenderness.

Q1. What is the most likely diagnosis?

Q2. What special tests could you use to help confirm the diagnosis?

Investigations

In order to support the clinical diagnosis, an MRI scan is requested (see Figure P5.1, below).

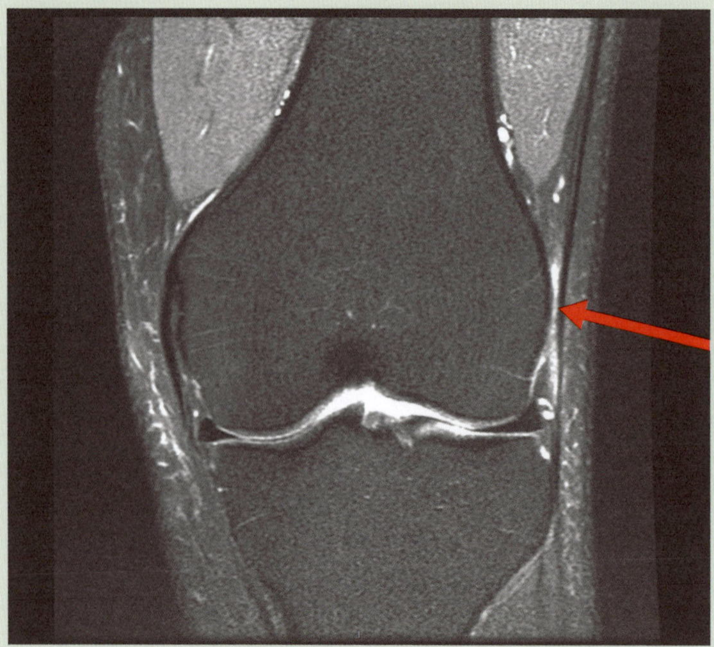

Q3. What does this image demonstrate?

Treatment

The cyclist is due to take part in a long-distance charity ride in six weeks' time. He would like to know more about his condition and get an idea of the likelihood of recovering in time.

Q4. What is the aetiology of his problem?

Q5. What treatment options are available?

Problem 5: Answers

Diagnosis: Iliotibial band (ITB) friction syndrome

A1. Iliotibial band friction syndrome.

A2. Ober's test may help to identify a tight iliotibial band. This test is performed with the patient lying on the unaffected side, with the hips flexed in order to straighten the lumbar lordosis. The leg is flexed 90° at the knee, while the examiner's hands stabilise the greater trochanter and hold up the ankle of the side being tested. The thigh is abducted passively and extended to catch the ITB over the greater trochanter. The thigh is then adducted passively. If the thigh remains suspended off the table, this indicates a shortened ITB.

In the Noble test, the patient is placed in a supine position with the knee at approximately 90° of flexion. Firm digital pressure is applied in the region of the lateral femoral epicondyle while the knee is passively extended. A positive result is pain elicited at approximately 30° of flexion over the lateral femoral epicondyle.

A3. The MRI demonstrates increased signal over the lateral femoral condyle and bursa underlying the ITB, suggesting localised inflammation. The MRI is also helpful in ruling out the differential diagnoses of meniscal or fibular collateral pathology.

A4. The condition is thought to arise due to repeated rubbing of the iliotibial band over the lateral femoral condyle in repetitive activities such as cycling and running. It may be due to training issues, abnormalities of the lower limb anatomy or muscle imbalance.

A5. In the acute phase, a protection, optimal loading, ice, compression and elevation (POLICE) regimen is followed by stretching of the ITB and the associated proximal musculature, i.e. the gluteus maximus and tensor facia latae. In runners, customised foot orthotics may be used to treat this condition by controlling the amount of inversion (medial rotation) of the foot, thus reducing rotation of the leg and knee. In cyclists, close attention should be paid to the set-up of the bike and the mechanics of the cyclist's pedalling. ITB compression wraps or taping may also be used. In cases where a conservative approach has failed, a steroid injection into the area may be helpful, and can be curative. Although controversial, surgical release of the ITB can be performed in severe, treatment-resistant cases.

4

Posterior structures

The popliteal fossa lies behind the knee joint, the joint itself being deeply placed in the fossa and forming part of the floor (see Figure 12, page 30). The remainder of the floor is formed proximally by the popliteal surface of the femur and distally by the posterior surface of the upper part of the tibia covered by the popliteus muscle (see Figures 13 and 16a, pages 30,33). The synovial membrane of the joint may herniate through the capsule, forming a swelling behind the knee known as a Baker's cyst (Figure 14, page 31).

The hamstring muscles descending from the thigh form its supero-lateral (biceps femoris) and supero-medial boundaries (semimembranosus and semitendinosus). As they descend to their insertions, they overlap the medial and lateral heads of the gastrocnemius muscle that form the infero-medial and infero-lateral boundaries respectively as they enter the calf. The lateral head often contains a small sesamoid bone, the fabella, which produces a characteristic image on a radiograph.

The popliteal fascia forms the roof of the fossa, investing the tendons and muscles like a bandage so that they are pulled nearer to the middle of the fossa and thus restrict the size of the roof. Traversing the fossa is the main blood and nerve supply to the leg and foot. Deepest, and entering from the medial side of the thigh through the adductor magnus hiatus, is the continuation of the femoral artery, which becomes the popliteal artery. It leaves the fossa and enters the leg beneath the soleal arch. It is relatively fixed at the points where it enters and leaves the fossa. Since it is deepest, and lies on the floor of the fossa, the artery is the most vulnerable to damage in dislocation of the knee.

The popliteal vein lies close to the artery but more superficial to it. Most superficial, descending from the posterior compartment of the thigh, just beneath the popliteal fascia, are the terminal branches of the sciatic nerve. The tibial nerve is the larger and bisects the fossa vertically as it descends to enter the calf deep to the soleus muscle. The common peroneal nerve passes infero-laterally beneath the tendon of the biceps femoris that it follows to reach the neck of the fibula.

The significant structures intimately associated with the posterior part of the capsule include the semimembranosus with its extensions and the popliteus muscle and its tendon as shown in Figures 16a and 16b on page 33.

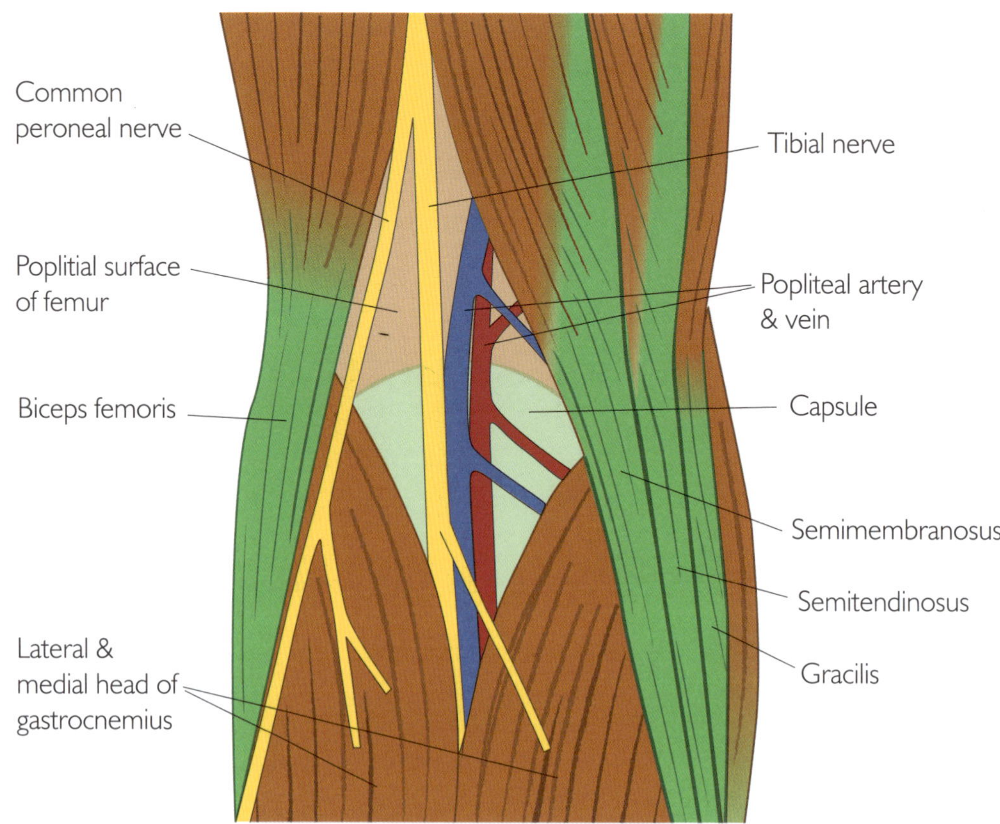

Figure 12: Knee posterior aspect showing popliteal fossa with boundaries and contents

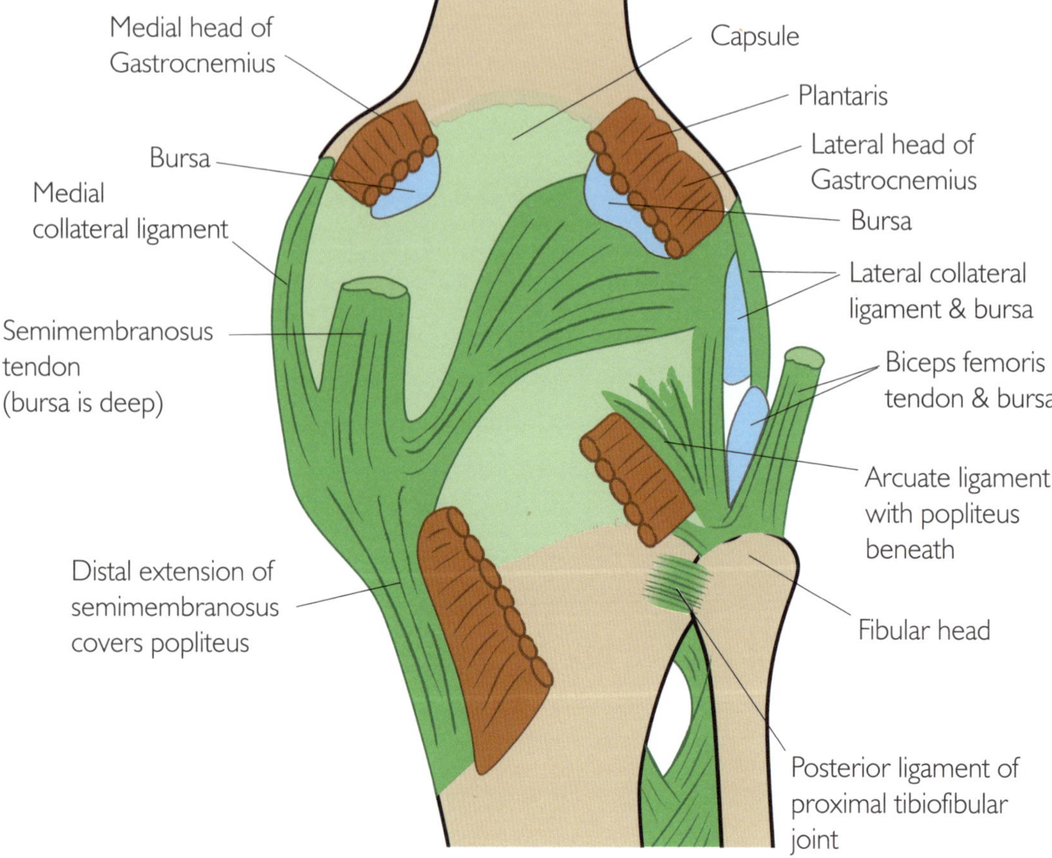

Figure 13: Posterior knee external features showing muscles, tendons with associated bursae, and ligaments

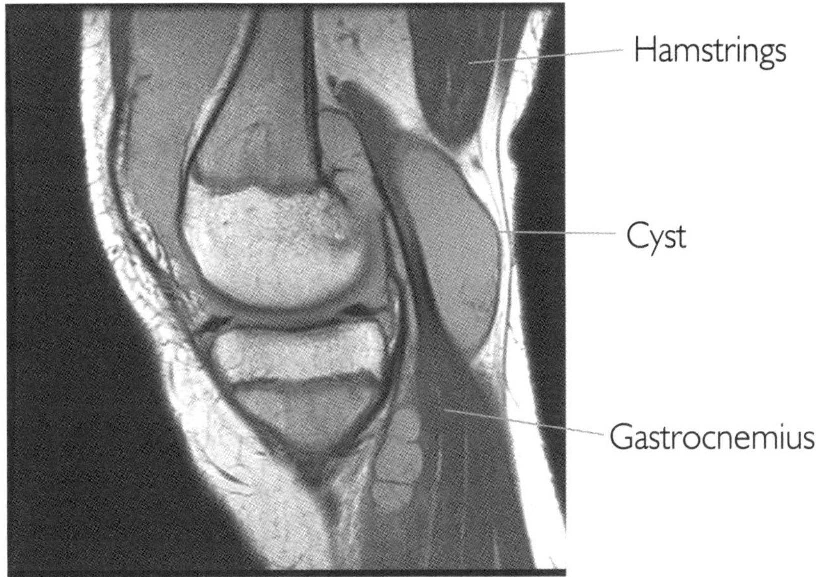

Figure 14: Sagittal MRI showing a Baker's cyst in a skeletally immature knee

The relationship of the popliteus tendon with the posterior aspect of the knee joint can be appreciated during arthroscopy whereby it is starkly visualised (see Figure 15). Popliteus tendinopathy can occur in athletes who frequently run around bends (e.g. 200m or 400m athletes), or on cambered surfaces (e.g. cross-country or fell runners). A popliteus muscle strain can also occur through a mechanism of forced leg rotation while the knee is flexed (Radhakrishna *et al.* 2004).

Problem 6

Sport – Sprinting in athletics

Clinical history

A 25-year-old male, national-level 200m sprinter complains of left (inside) leg posterolateral knee pain. It has come on gradually over the last four weeks when he has been completing more than usual repetitions of bend running practice in preparation for an upcoming championship. He cannot recall an injurious event and denies that he has any symptoms of catching, locking or knee swelling. Initially the discomfort was mild and went away following his warm-up. However, it is now present throughout his sessions, limiting his ability to 'attack' the bend. The athlete also complains of posterior knee stiffness and soreness with terminal extension for the first 30 minutes after rising the day after track training sessions. There are no mechanical symptoms.

Q1. What structures might be the source of the athlete's pain?

Examination

Examination of the runner's knee revealed tenderness deep in the posterolateral corner of the knee. There was no effusion or instability, and meniscal provocation tests were negative.

Q2. How could pain on contraction of each of the posterolateral knee tendons be tested?

Investigations

Plain x-rays of the athlete's knee have been performed and these were reported to be 'normal'.

Q3. Which imaging modality might best differentiate knee joint or meniscal pathology from posterolateral knee soft tissue injury?

Treatment

MRI confirms inflammation in the region of the popliteus tendon.

Q4. What is the aetiology of his problem?

Q5. What treatment options are available?

Problem 6: Answers

Diagnosis: Popliteus tendinopathy

A1. a. Popliteus tendon.

b. Biceps femoris distal tendinopathy/enesopathy.

c. Posterolateral corner capsular or ligamentous strain.

d. Posterolateral meniscal derangement.

e. Posterolateral knee osteo-chondral derangement.

A2. a. Biceps femoris – resisted knee flexion with the tibia held in slight external rotation.

b. Popliteus – resisted knee flexion in Figure 4 position.

A3. Magnetic resonance imaging.

A4. Popliteal tendinopathy is due to repetitive strain on the tendon as it acts in its outer range whilst the inside leg tibia is relatively externally rotated during bend runs.

A5. In the acute phase, the POLICE regimen and modification of training techniques, including a period of reduction or avoidance of bend running, may reduce the symptoms. Oral anti-inflammatory drugs may be of some help, as may an ultrasound guided local injection.

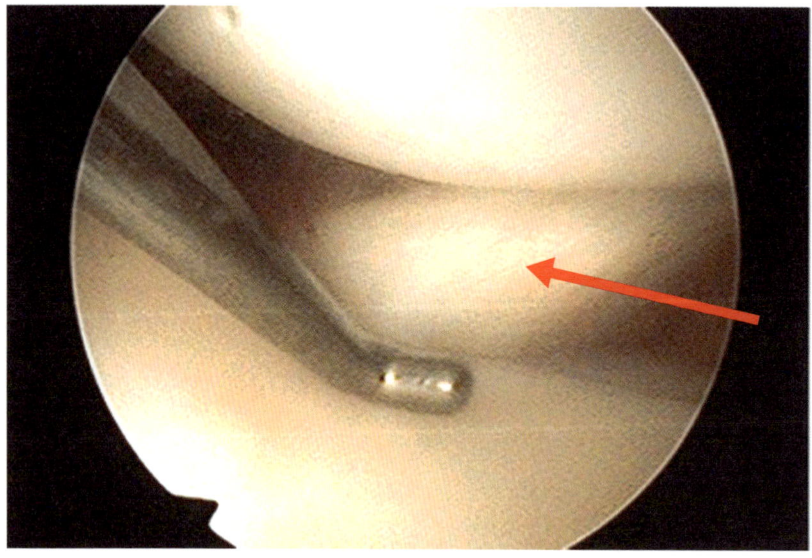

Figure 15: Arthroscopy of normal popliteus tendon (right knee)

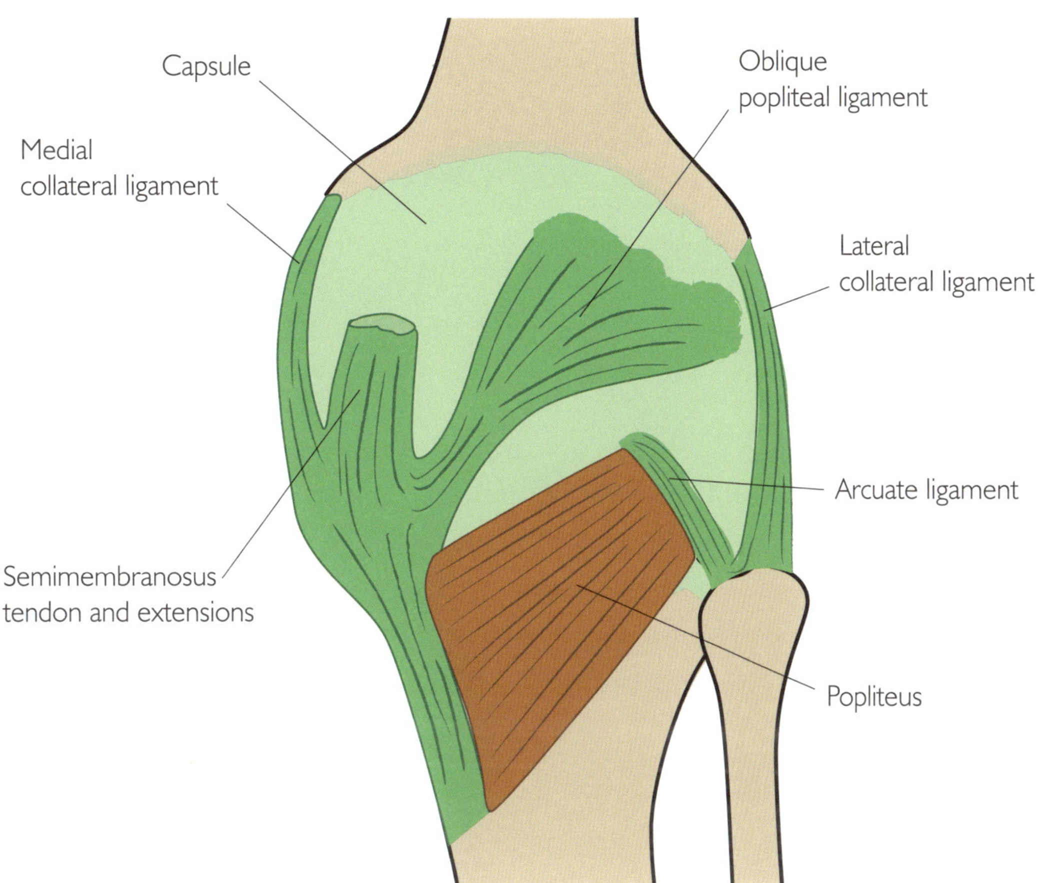

Figure 16a: Posterior knee external features: muscles, tendons and associated ligaments

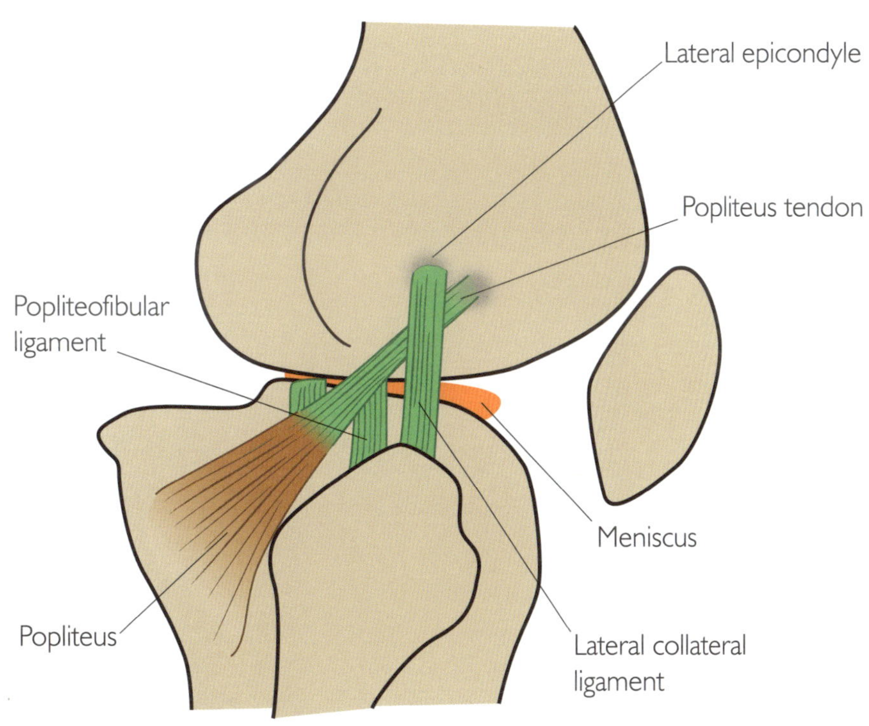

Figure 16b: Posterolateral knee features. The capsule has been removed.

Problem 7

Sport – Rugby

Clinical history

A 24-year-old man was playing professional rugby. He was jumping to avoid an opponent on the ground when he landed on his right leg. At that moment an opposing player slid in forcing his knee into a varus position. The player 'felt something go' at the outside of his knee and had to leave the field.

Q1. What is the most likely diagnosis?

Q2. What is the most appropriate initial management?

Examination

Examination of the knee revealed a small effusion. There was swelling around the posterolateral corner of the knee. The patient complained of some numbness in the foot during the examination but there was no evidence of weakness of dorsiflexion or plantar flexion of the ankle. The knee was unstable to varus testing. There was no evidence of antero-posterior laxity.

Q3. What structures that make up the posterolateral corner of the knee may have been damaged?

Q4. Why might the patient complain of numbness in the foot?

Investigations

A plain x-ray (see Figure P7.1) and an MRI scan (see Figures P7.2 and P7.3) are arranged.

Q5. What do these investigations demonstrate?

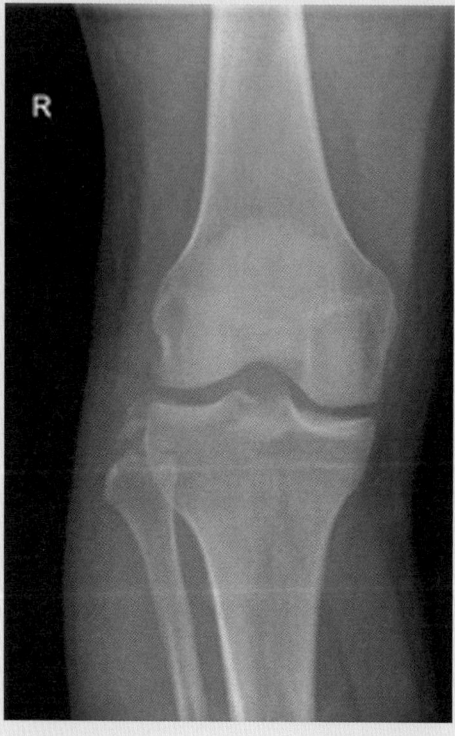

Figure P7.1 Coronal knee x-radiograph

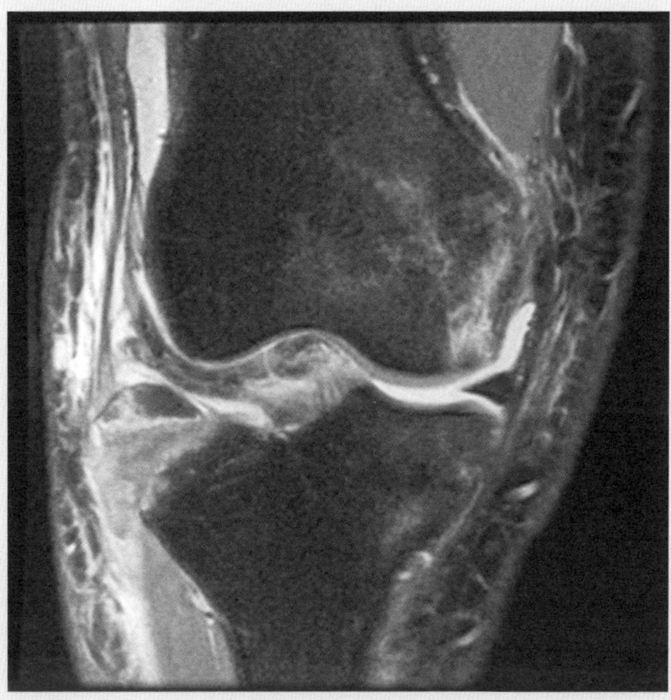

Figure P7.2: Coronal knee MRI

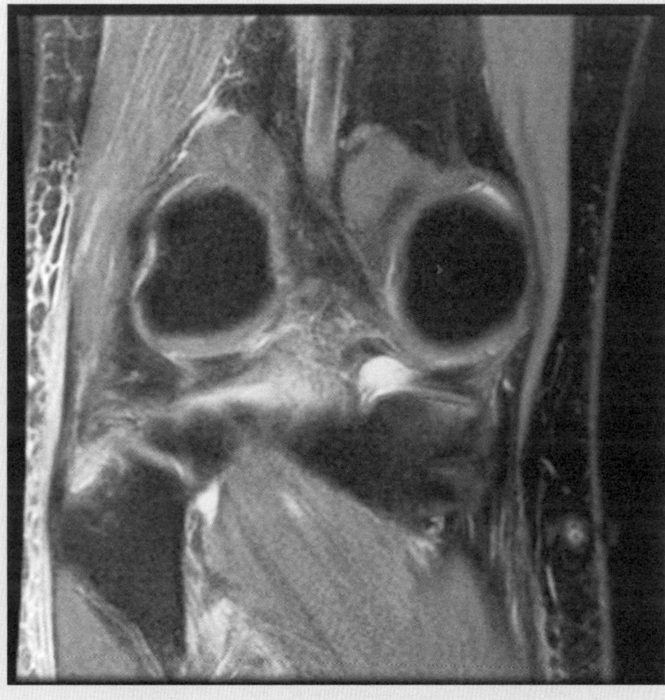

Figure P7.3: Coronal knee MRI

Treatment

The player tells you that he is hoping to continue his rugby career.

Q6. What treatment options are available and what is the prognosis for the player being able to return to rugby?

Problem 7: Answers

Diagnosis: Posterolateral corner injury

A1. a. Posterolateral corner injury.
b. Anterior cruciate injury.

A2 a. POLICE regimen, including splinting and provision of crutches to protect the injured structures from further damage.
b. Neurological and vascular assessment of the leg.
c. Transfer to a medical facility.

A3. a. Fibular (lateral) collateral ligament.
b. Biceps femoris tendon.
c. Popliteus.
d. Lateral joint capsule.
e. Lateral meniscus.

A4. The patient is likely to have sustained a traction neuropraxia injury to the common peroneal nerve as it winds around the fibular neck.

A5. The plain x-ray (see Figure P7.1) demonstrates an avulsion fracture of the fibular head and evidence of damage to the antero-lateral tibial plateau. MRI scans (see Figures P7.2 and P7.3) confirm this.

A6. In order to prevent long-term instability, surgical reconstruction is indicated (see Figures P7.4 and P7.5). It is important at the time of surgery that the common peroneal nerve is visualised and explored in particular if there is evidence of neurological compromise.

A return to professional rugby may be possible. The prognosis for a prolonged return would be less positive if:

- Any neuropraxia persists
- There is any misalignment of the fixated tibial plateau that might predispose to articular cartilage damage
- There is significant ongoing functional instability of the lateral knee.

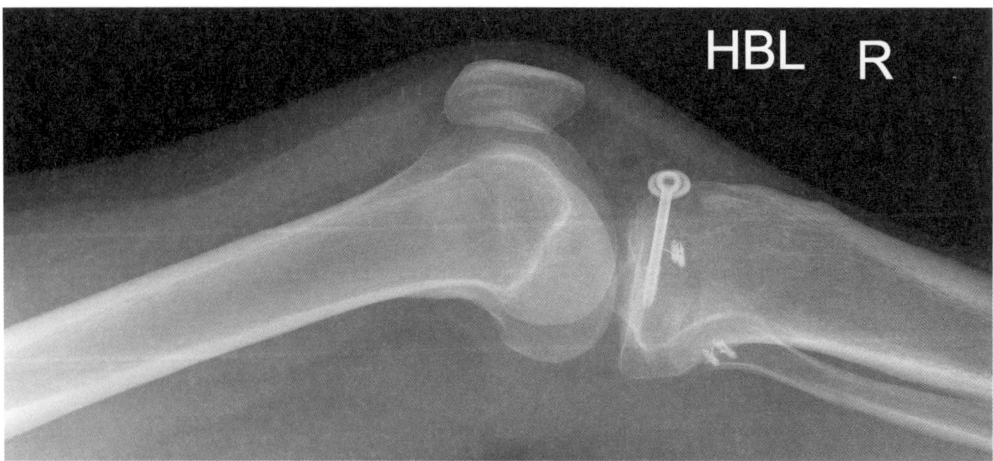

Figure P7.4

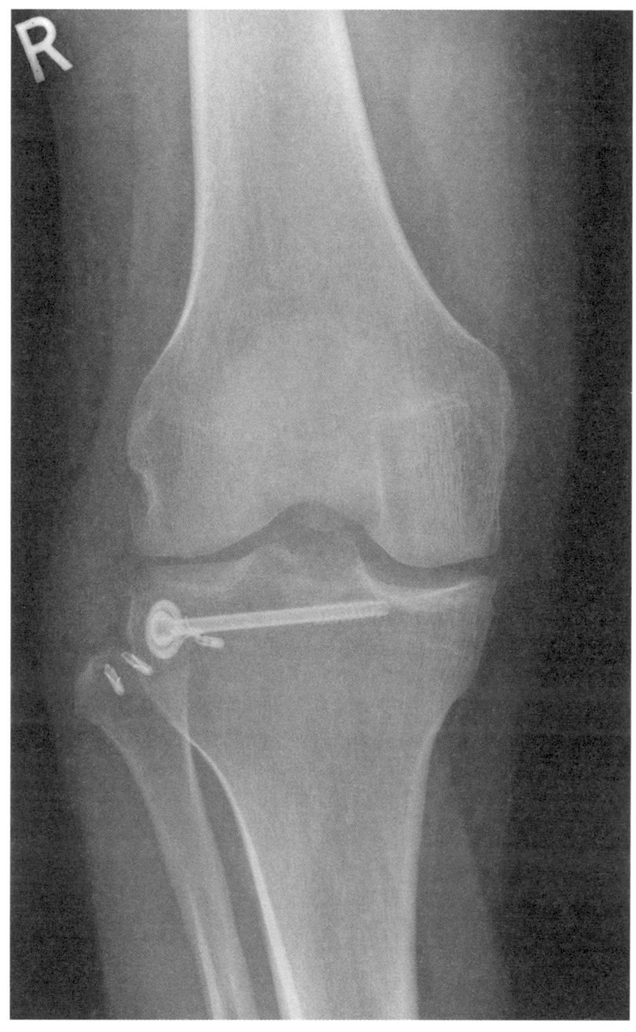

Figure P7.5

5

Medial structures

The tendons of sartorius, gracilis and semitendinosus form a triad as they descend towards the tibia. There they fuse together and form a layered attachment called the pes anserinus ('goose's foot') on the upper anterior subcutaneous surface of the tibia, immediately below the medial condyle (see Figure 17). A bursa lies beneath it and may present clinically as bursitis.

The medial collateral ligament forms a thick band in the joint capsule, passing from the medial epicondyle of the femur down to the tibial condyle. The medial patellar retinaculum passes from the medial border of the patella backwards towards the collateral ligament. The tendon of the semimembranosus is the most posterior structure descending to the tibial condyle and has an important role in stabilising the posteromedial side of the joint. Finally the lower fibres of the vastus medialis are conspicuous on the upper medial side of the knee as they pass to be attached to the medial border of the patella.

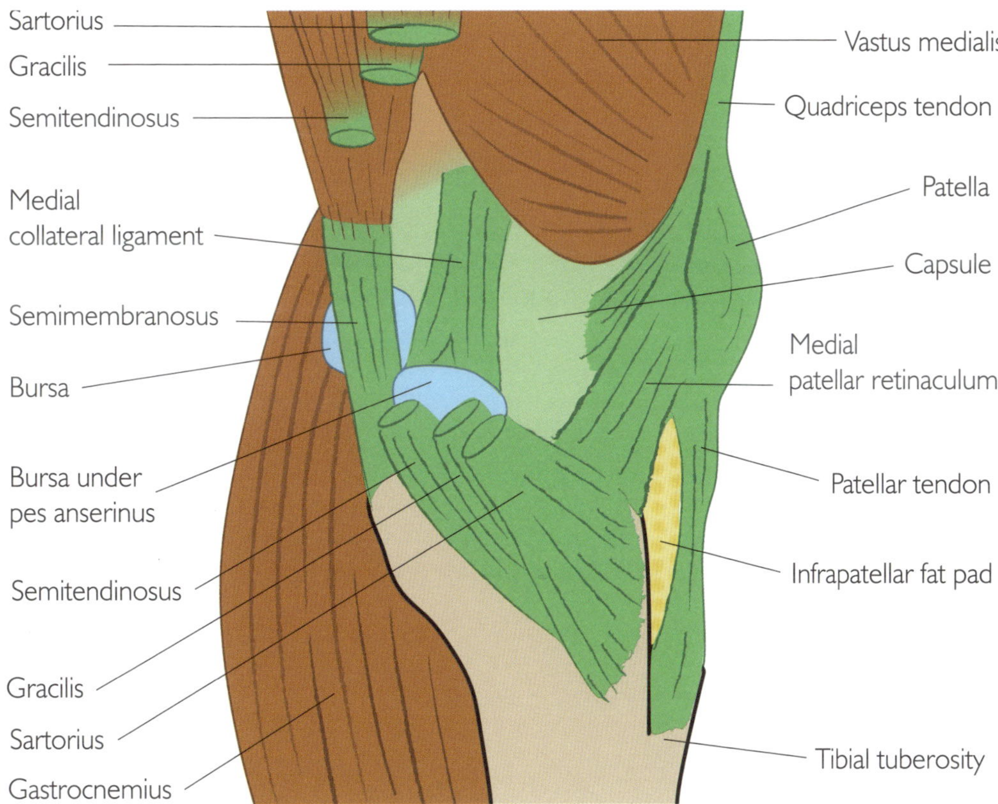

Figure 17: Medial knee external features: muscles, tendons with associated bursae, and ligaments

6

Lateral structures

Iliotibial band (ITB)

The iliotibial band is a long, thickened band in the fascia lata of the thigh, which descends lateral to the knee to attach to a flat facet on the front of the lateral tibial condyle, close to the tibial tuberosity (see Figure 19 and also Figure 51, page 74). Lying in front of the transverse axis of the joint, it is tensed by the gluteus maximus and tensor fasciae latae and has an important role in keeping the knee extended when standing in a fully upright position. As the knee is flexed, the band travels posteriorly across the epicondyle (see Figure 18).

Pain felt over the posterolateral part of the knee, together with local tenderness over the lateral femoral condyle, may be associated with iliotibial band friction syndrome. This syndrome is especially seen in runners, particularly those traversing cambered surfaces and those performing repeated bends during training. It is also common in cyclists (Ferber *et al.* 2010).

Fairclough *et al.* (2006) found the iliotibial band (ITB) was compressed against the lateral epicondyle at 30° knee flexion consequent to tibial internal rotation (Fairclough *et al.* 2006; Toumi *et al.* 2006). They suggest that the pain associated with the ITB syndrome may be due to compression of a richly innervated and vascularised collection of fat lying under the band as it rolls over the epicondyle during knee flexion. There was no evidence of a bursa beneath the ITB in the region of the knee. However, Lobenhoffer *et al.* (1996) found nociceptive sensory endings to be particularly concentrated in the tibial attachment of the ITB.

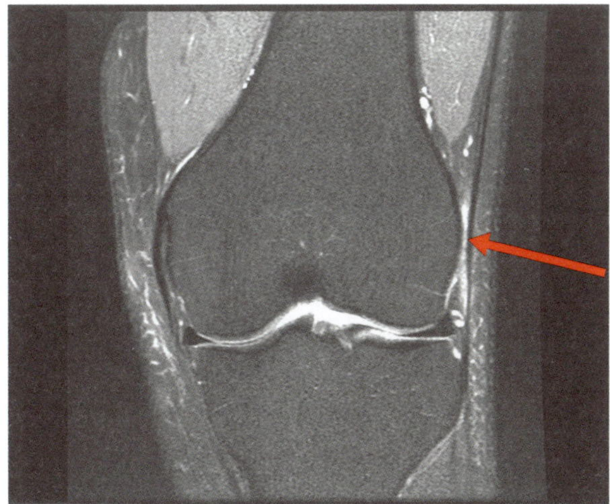

Figure 18: Iliotibial band friction syndrome
The red arrow marks the thin dark line of the ilio-tibial band as it crosses the lateral epicondyle of the femur. The white area of high signal deep to the band indicates oedema associated with ilio-tibial band friction syndrome.

The lateral collateral ligament is a cord-like thickening in the capsule that extends from the epicondyle of the femur to the styloid process on the head of the fibula.

The tendon of the biceps is a conspicuous posterior structure passing downwards to its attachment on the styloid process of the fibula. Here it overlies and obscures the lateral collateral ligament. The lateral patella retinaculum passes from the lateral border of the patella towards the collateral ligament. The common peroneal nerve descends from the popliteal fossa under cover of the biceps femoris to reach the head of the fibula below. The common peroneal nerve then winds forwards around the neck of the fibula, where it enters the peroneus longus. In this part of its course the nerve is vulnerable to compression and to fracture of the fibula.

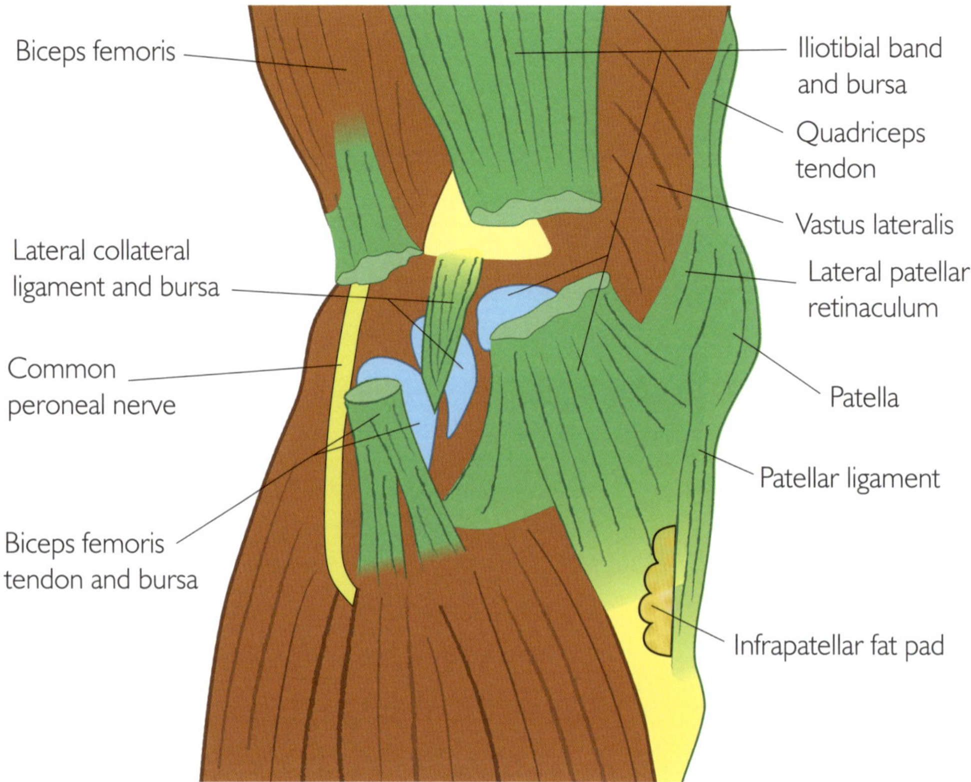

Figure 19: Lateral knee external features: muscles, ligaments, tendons and associated bursae

Note: the presence of a bursa beneath the iliotibial band (see Figure 19) is disputed by some investigators (Fairclough *et al.* 2007).

7

Blood supply

The knee joint has a substantial blood supply from branches of the femoral, profunda femoris, popliteal, posterior and anterior tibial arteries. The popliteal artery itself is vulnerable to damage, as in dislocation (Robertson *et al.* 2006). This is because the popliteal artery is relatively fixed proximally where it passes through the hiatus in adductor magnus. It is also fairly fixed distally where it passes beneath the soleal arch into the leg. Consequently it cannot tolerate much distortion.

These arteries form an extensive genicular anastomosis on all sides of the joint (see Figure 20). In particular, a middle genicular branch (see also Figure 56, page 77) arises from the popliteal artery and penetrates the posterior part of the capsule to supply the cruciate ligaments. It may be damaged if these ligaments are torn. The main purpose of the anastomosis is to provide a rich blood supply to the capsule and particularly to the synovial membrane lining the capsule. The anastomosis also provides an alternative route for blood flow into the leg and foot in the event of obstruction of the distal part of the femoral or of the popliteal artery, but this can be regarded as incidental.

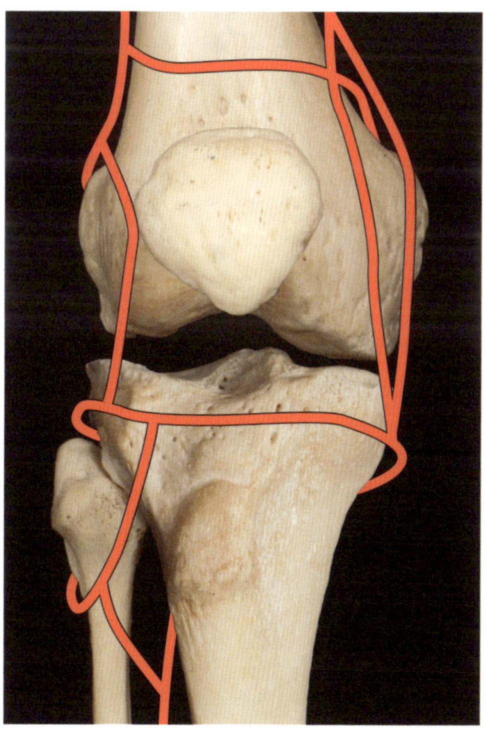

Figure 20: Genicular anastomosis

8

Synovial membrane and synovial fluid

Synovial membrane lines the inside of the capsule and non-articular structures, including the infrapatellar fat pad, popliteus tendon and cruciate ligaments, which invaginate the membrane. This synovial membrane is extensive, particularly in relation to the distal end of the femur (see Figure 21). It has an extremely rich capillary network, fed from the genicular anastomosis, and the structure of the membrane facilitates easy transfer of fluid from the capillaries into the synovial cavity during the formation of synovial fluid (Horky 1981).

It must be emphasised that there is a *dynamic turnover of synovial fluid* (Levick & McDonald 1995), which occurs within the span of 24 hours, and this has important clinical implications. Thus, capillary dilation and concomitant increased permeability (which may accompany trauma to the knee joint) result in increased production of synovial fluid. This fluid accumulates in the joint as an effusion, since the lymphatics draining the joint are overwhelmed by the increase. Further evidence of capillary dilation is provided by redness and warmth in the skin over the joint when it is acutely inflamed.

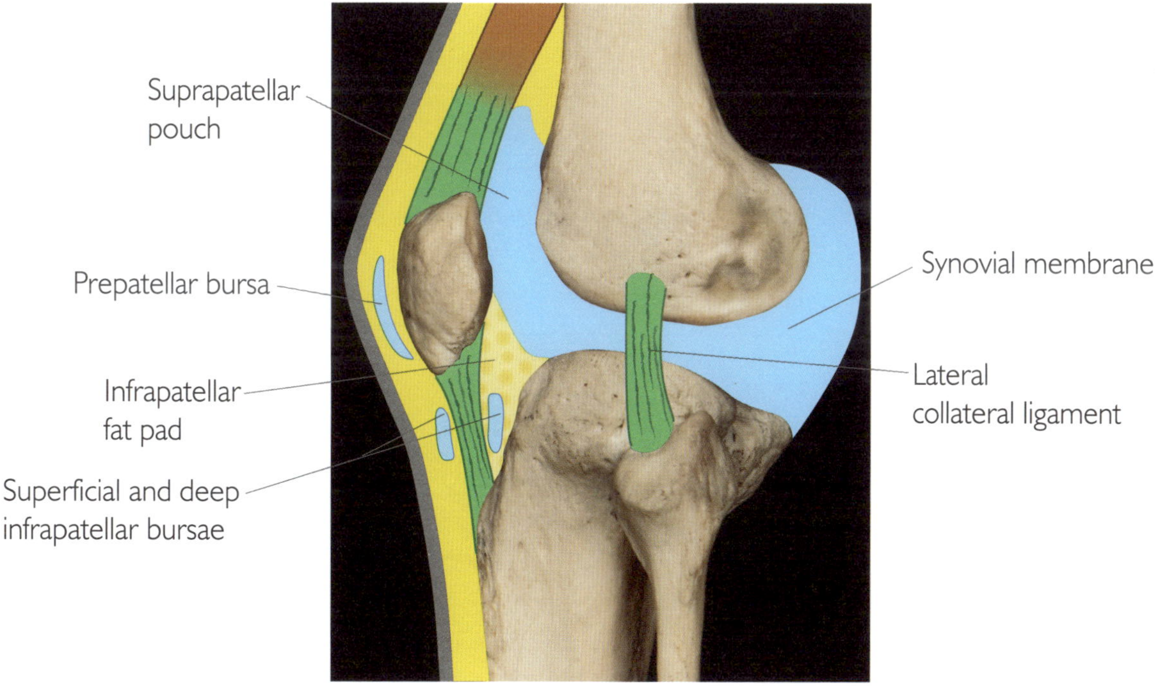

Figure 21: Knee joint synovial membrane and anterior bursae (cruciate ligaments and capsule not shown)

Medio-patellar plica

An infolding (plica) of the synovial membrane into the interior of the joint on the medial side extends from the suprapatellar pouch downwards behind the patella to be continuous inferiorly with the synovia lining the infrapatellar fat pad (see Figures 22a and 22b). The infolding may extend so deeply into the joint that it lies between the medial facet of the patella and the medial femoral condyle (Garcia-Valtuille *et al.* 2002). It may be the remains of an intercondylar septum in the foetus, which divided the joint vertically into two halves. In sports such as running and cycling, which involve repetitive flexion and extension of the knee, the plica may become trapped as it passes between the facet of the patella and the medial femoral condyle (Garcia-Valtuille *et al.* 2002). This causes the plica to become inflamed and may lead to swelling and pain along the medial border of the patella.

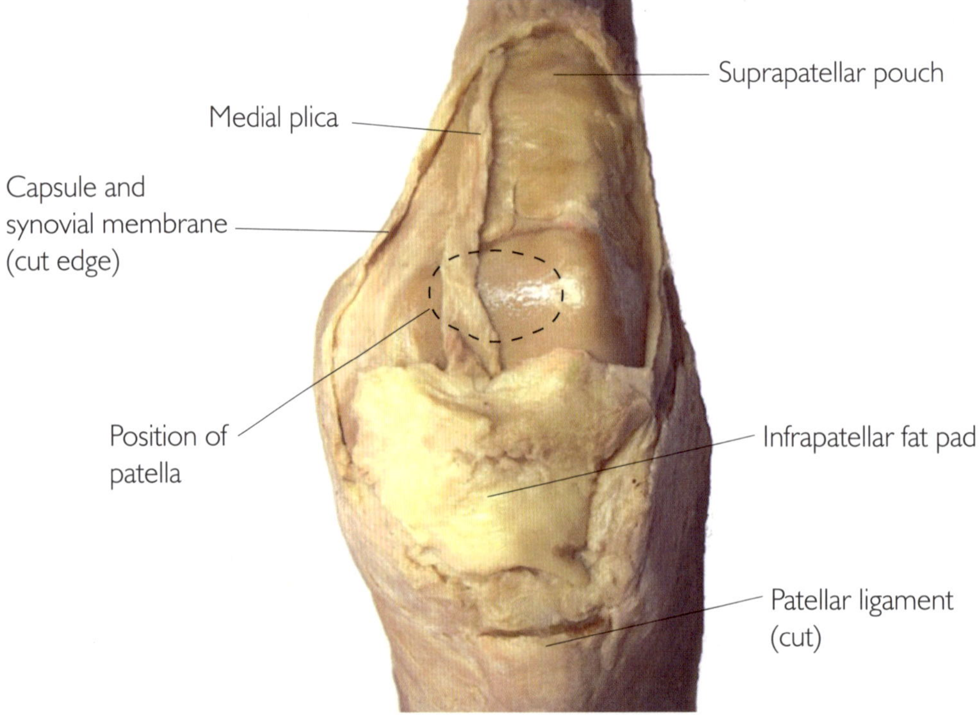

Figure 22a: Patella and anterior part of capsule removed to show plica

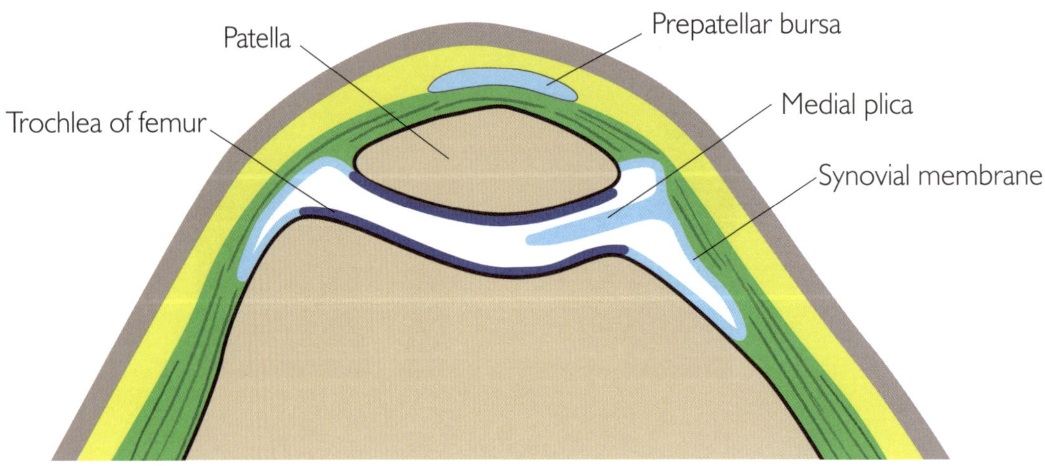

Figure 22b: Transverse section through suprapatellar bursa to show medial plica

Bursae

There are numerous bursae around the knee joint that are located anteriorly, posteriorly and on each side (see Figures 21, 22b, 25, 26 and 27). They are lined by synovial membrane and are thought to prevent excessive friction between structures lying near the joint and the capsule itself, especially ligaments and tendons where they attach close to the capsule. Most of the bursae do not communicate with the main synovial cavity of the knee joint, but some do – including the large suprapatellar bursa lying antero-superiorly and also the bursa for the semimembranosus tendon posteriorly.

In sports injuries, bursae may become inflamed (bursitis) as a result of direct trauma over the bursa or adjacent soft tissues. Other causes include repeated or prolonged pressure over the bursa, and constant overuse of overlying muscles and tendons with associated friction on the bursa. The bursitis is shown by pain and swelling. In knee joint effusions, fluid may collect in the suprapatellar pouch and this forms the basis of the patellar tap test. A Baker's cyst (see Figure 14, page 31), which appears posteriorly in the popliteal fossa, is a herniation of the synovial membrane through the capsule and may enlarge progressively. It resembles a bursa but is not classified as such.

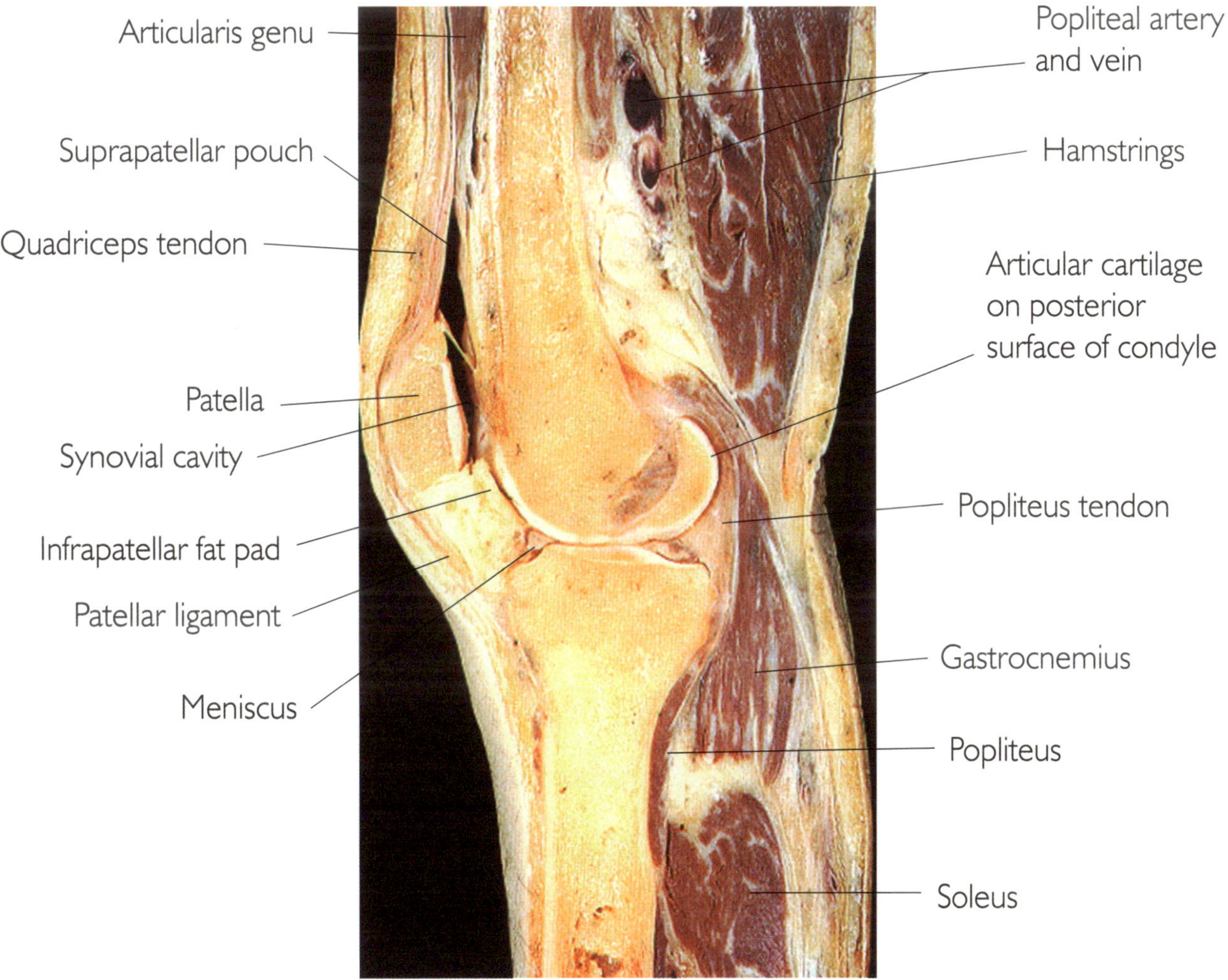

Figure 23: Sagittal section through the knee (medial compartment)

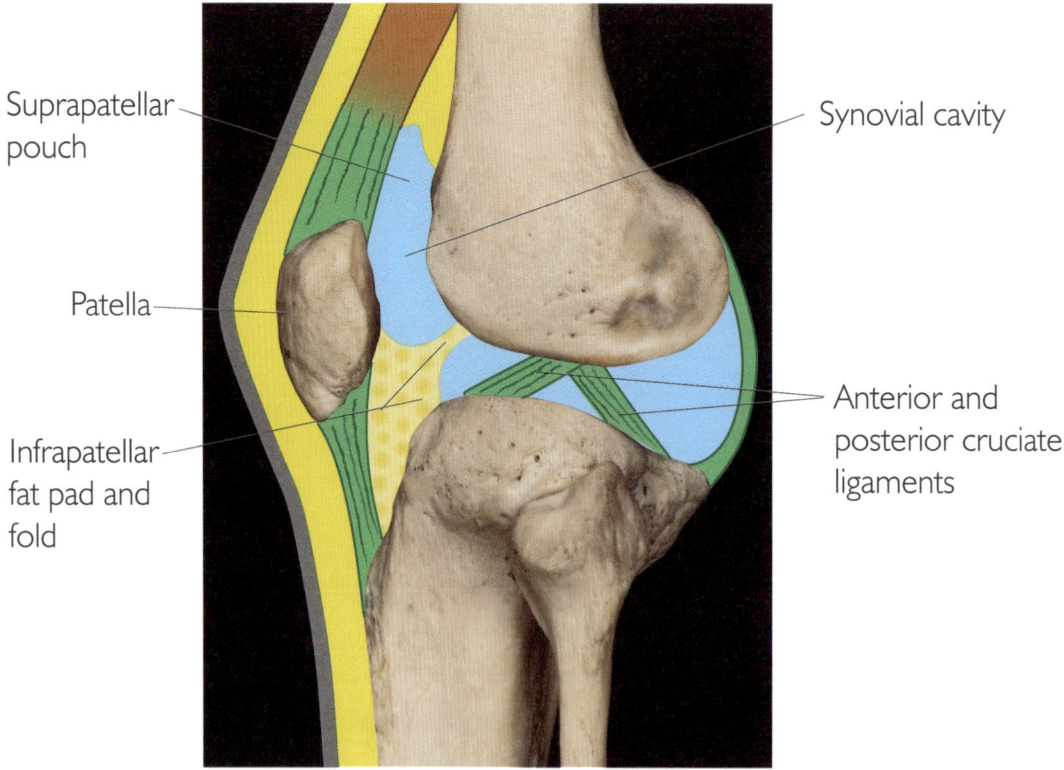

Figure 24: Knee joint sagittal section

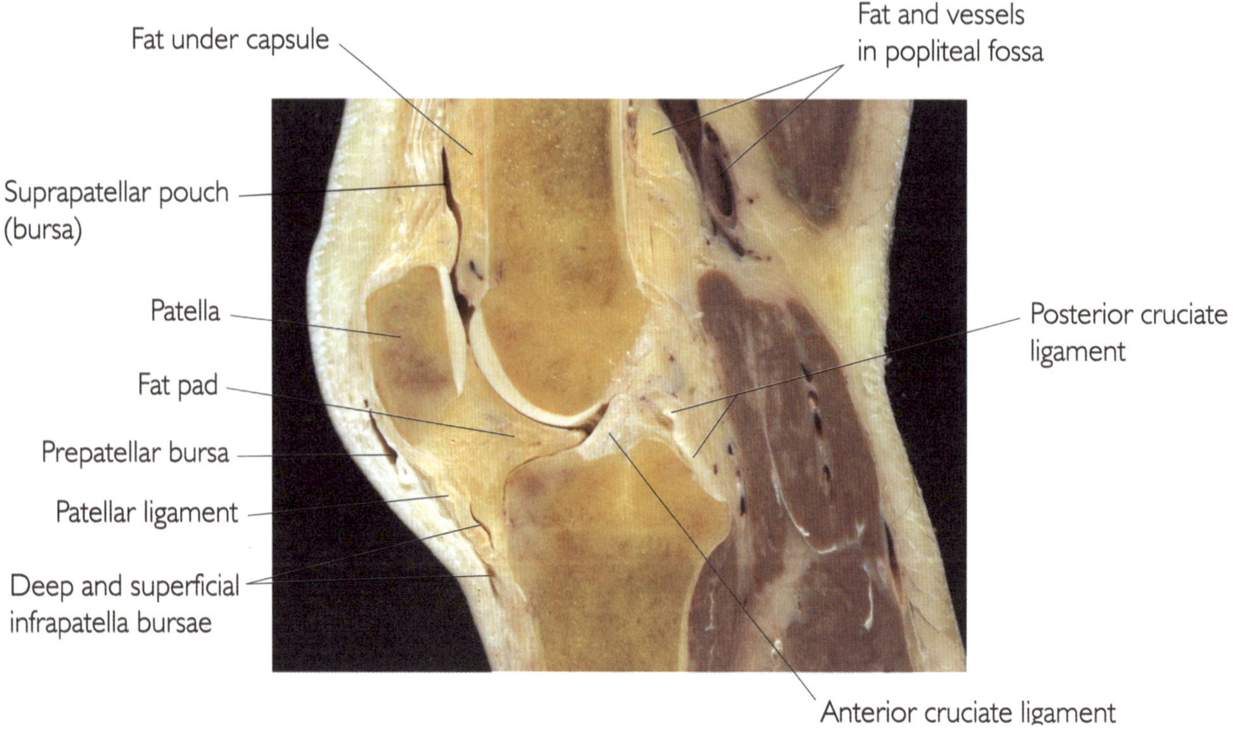

Figure 25: Sagittal section of knee showing anterior bursae

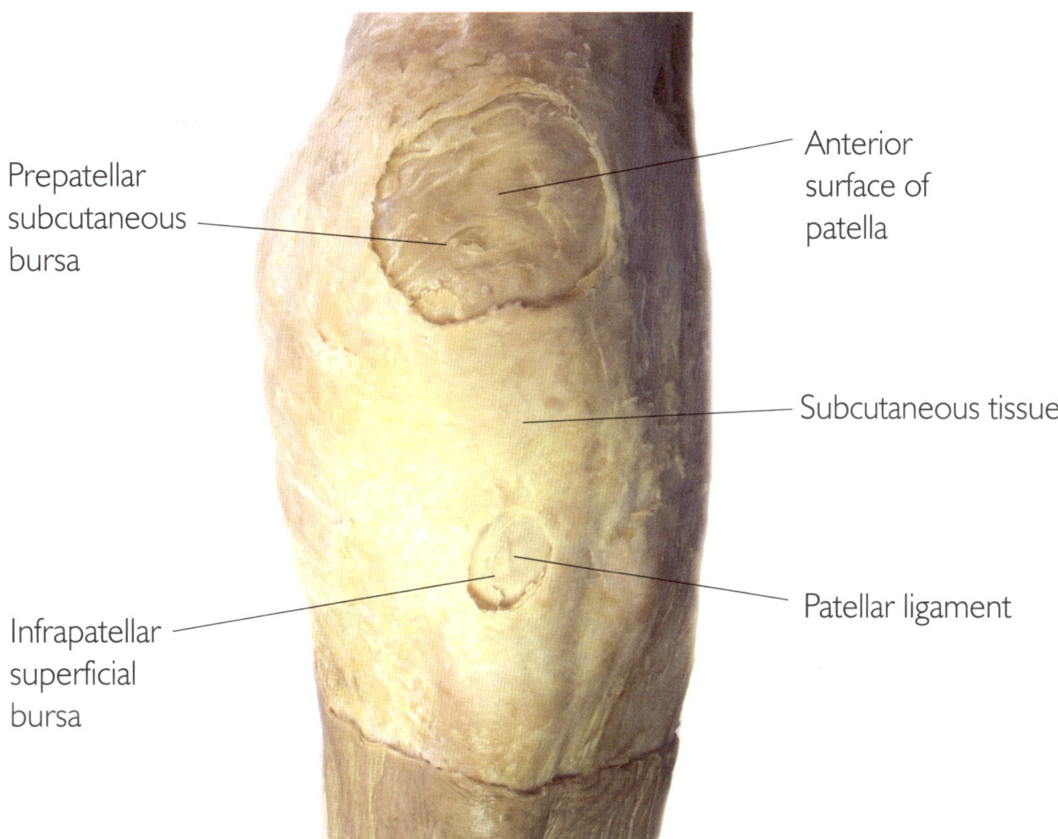

Figure 26: Anterior subcutaneous bursae of the knee

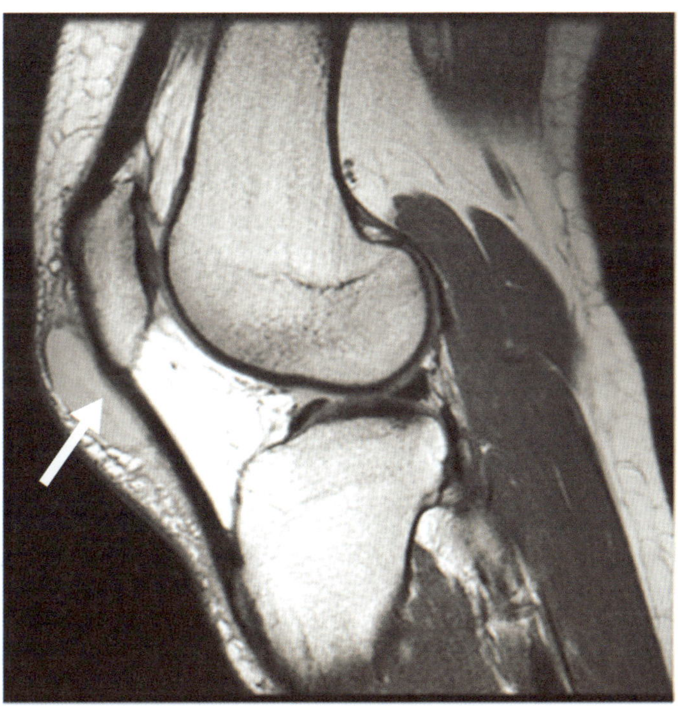

Figure 27: Sagittal MRI of knee showing prepatellar bursitis (white arrow)

9

Major intra-articular structures

The major structures within the knee joint that are of particular concern to sports practitioners are the medial and lateral meniscus and the two cruciate ligaments (Figure 28). The menisci may be torn by trauma or affected by degenerative changes and the ligaments may sustain partial or complete (rupture) strain injuries.

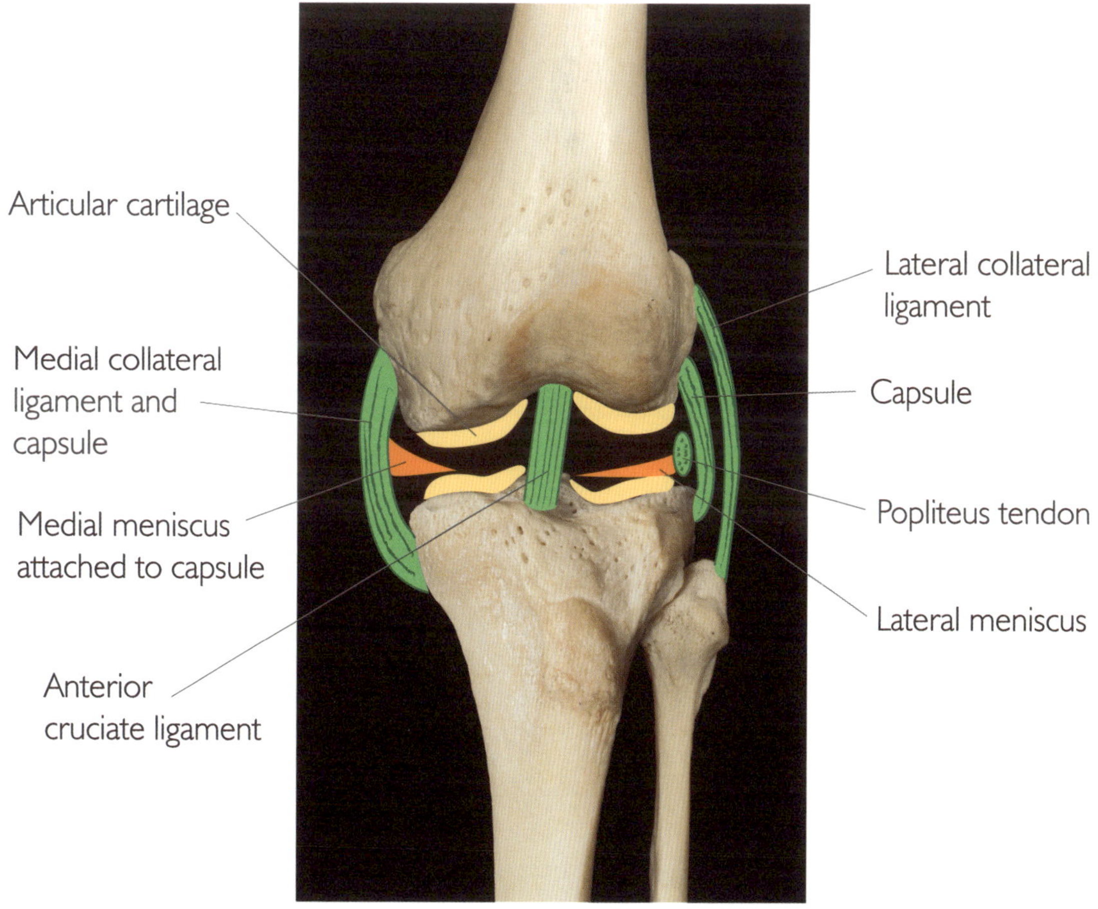

Figure 28: Diagram of knee joint coronal section

Menisci

The two menisci, medial and lateral, lie interposed between the respective condyles of the femur and tibia and are in contact with the articular cartilage of the condyles. They are crescent- or C-shaped (see Figures 29 and 34, page 55) and composed of fibrocartilage. Their upper surfaces are concave and articulate with the femoral condyles, whilst their inferior surfaces are flat and articulate with the tibial condyles (see Figure 30). Their lateral borders are convex and attached to the fibrous capsule by thickenings called coronary ligaments (see Figure 47, page 69). Their inner borders are concave and free.

The medial meniscal cartilage has the form of a more open C compared with the lateral. The lateral also has a larger surface area (see Figure 29), both factors being significant regarding their respective functions (see page 54). In cross-section they are wedge shaped, being thick on their lateral border but thin on their inner border. The tips of each meniscus (horns) are attached by fibrous bands to the medial or lateral tubercles on the intercondylar eminence of the tibia. Meniscotibial (coronary) ligaments (see Figures 46 and 47, pages 67,69) stabilise the lateral borders.

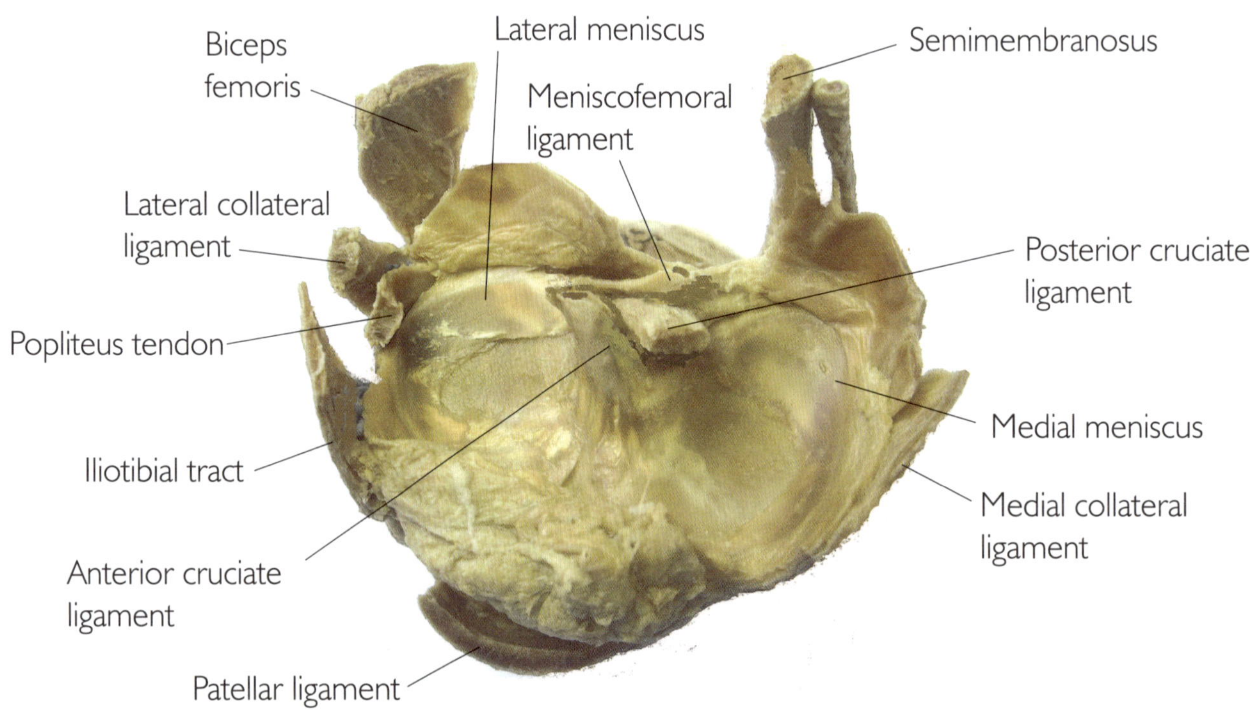

Figure 29: Tibial plateau with menisci, cruciate ligaments and related adjacent ligaments and tendons viewed from above

Figure 30 shows a frontal view of the interior of the knee joint. The patella has been removed, together with the infrapatellar fat pad. Note that the medial collateral ligament is attached to the adjacent medial meniscus but the lateral meniscus is not attached to the adjacent collateral ligament.

Menisci are not completely avascular. Small blood vessels enter the peripheral (thicker) part of the meniscus from the capsule (see Figures 31 and 32). The inner (thinner) part is avascular. This has important implications for possible healing of torn menisci (Arnoczky & Warren 1982).

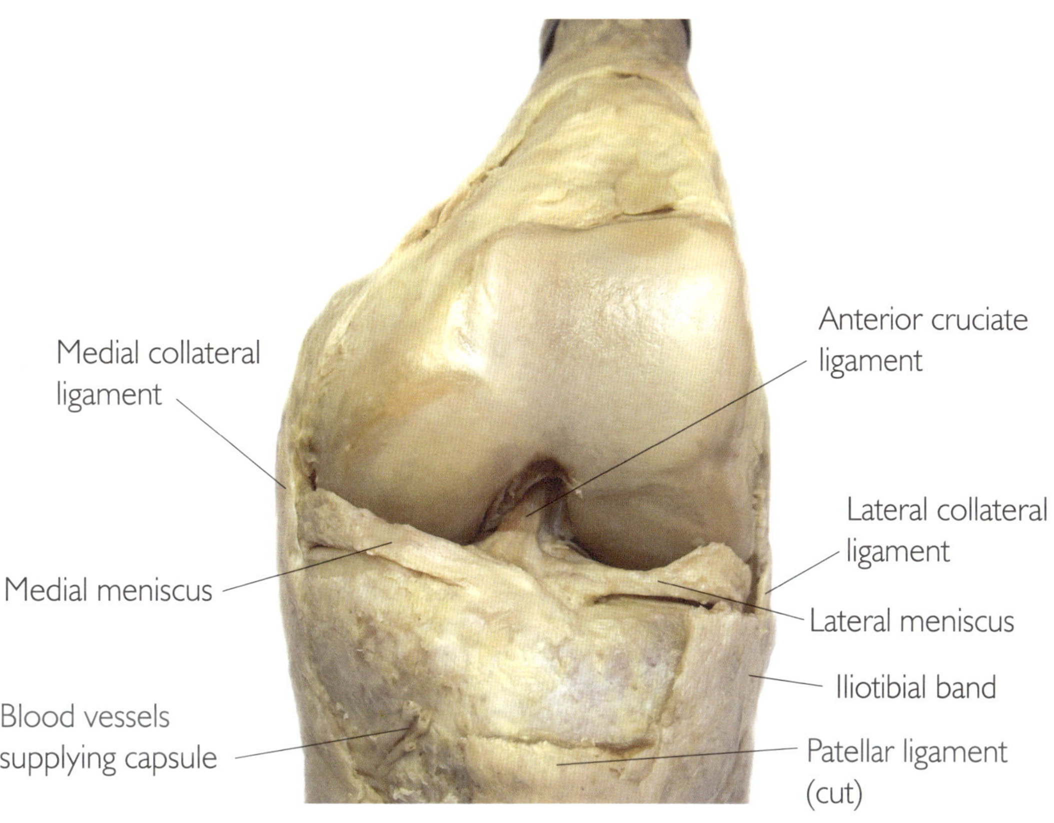

Figure 30: Frontal view of interior of knee joint.

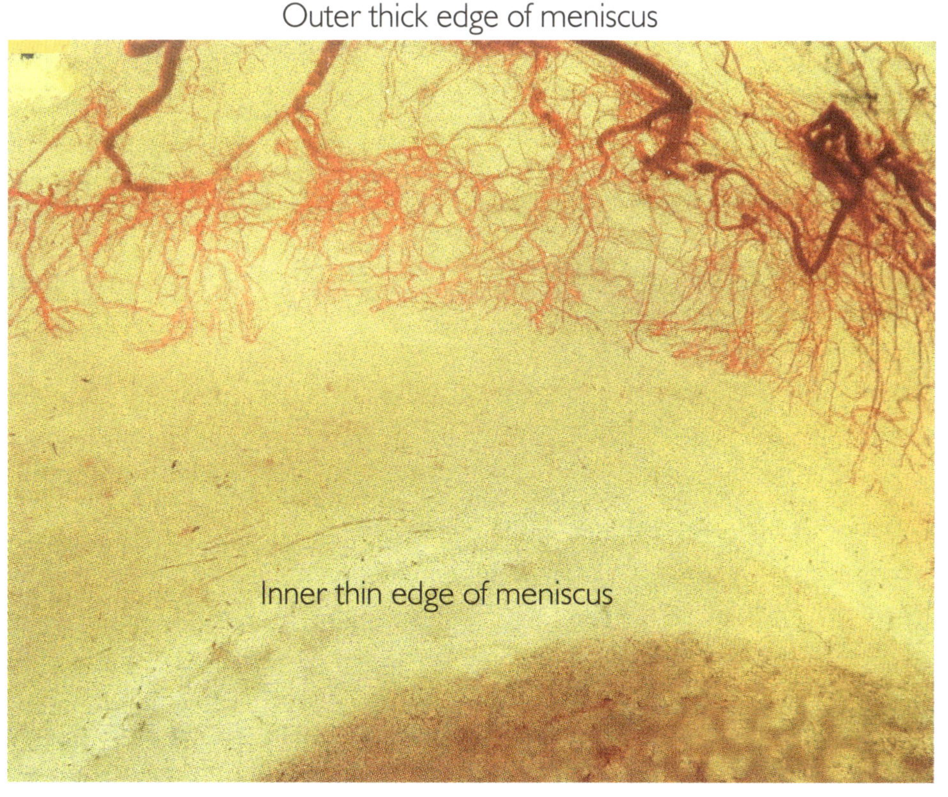

Figure 31: Blood vessels in the peripheral part of the meniscus

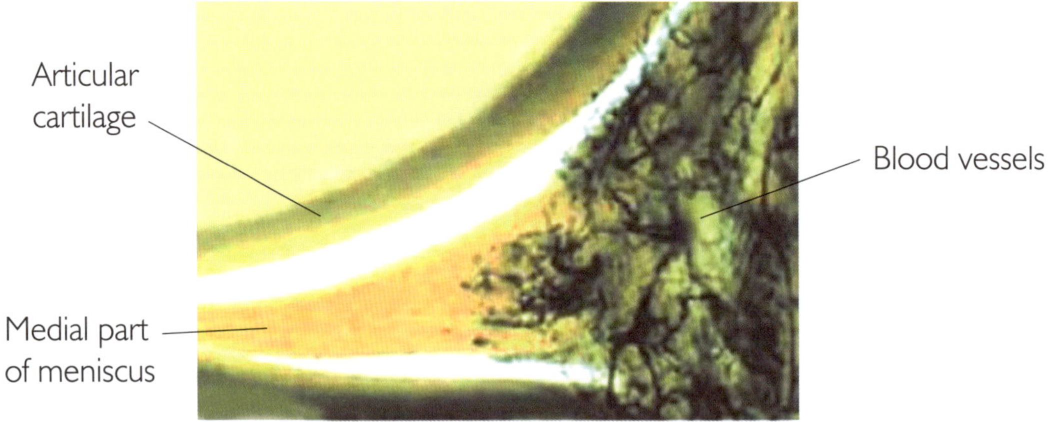

Figure 32: Blood supply to peripheral 'red zone' of meniscus that may be amenable to repair if torn

Overall, the medial meniscus is larger and thicker than the lateral, which is smaller, flatter and embraced within the horns of the medial cartilage. This reflects their differing functions in movements of the joint. In the medial compartment, the major movement between the respective femoral and tibial condyles is flexion or extension (hinge), together with some pivoting. In the lateral compartment, not only is there hinge and pivot movement but also significant gliding, the meniscus being held by the meniscofemoral ligament firmly under the femoral condyle whilst they both glide on the tibial plateau during completion of extension. In general, there is greater movement of the menisci in relation to the tibia than to the femur, and more movement of the lateral as compared with the medial meniscus. Also, both menisci move slightly forward during extension and backward in flexion.

The four main functions of the knee menisci are:

1. Transmission of load (50–70%); the posterior horns carry more load than the anterior horns; reduction of stress (load per unit area)
2. Shock absorption, protecting the underlying hyaline cartilage and subchondral bone
3. Assisting lubrication and therefore nutrition of cartilage
4. Increasing the congruity (fit) of the articulating surfaces.

Meniscal disorders

Meniscal tears

Menisci may become torn, particularly when subjected to torsion stresses together with vertical compression, resulting in shearing force (see Figure 33). They may also be damaged during hyperflexion or hyperextension. The medial meniscus is five times more likely to be damaged than the lateral. The lateral meniscus is, however, most likely to be damaged in conjunction with an acute anterior cruciate ligament injury.

Meniscal tears are generally classified by their morphology. The tears may split the meniscus radially or circumferentially. The types of tear and their progression are shown in Figures 34a and 34b on pages 55,56. They can be readily visualised by MRI (see Figure 35, page 56) and by arthroscopy (see Figures 36 and 37, page 56,59). The radial tear may enlarge and result in a flap that intrudes into the joint cavity. The vertical tear may enlarge and develop into a 'bucket handle'. This 'bucket handle' may swing and prolapse into the interior of the joint, where it may impact between the articulating surfaces, causing locking of the joint. Vertical (circumferential) tears more commonly result from direct trauma in younger patients.

Early identification of these tears is crucial, as – unlike most radial tears – they may be amenable to repair as a result of their occurrence in the vascular zone of the meniscus. A chronically displaced meniscal tear may become plastically deformed as a result of being loaded during weight-bearing and become irreducible. If a total or near total meniscectomy is required, particularly in the lateral compartment, the increased load transmission to the articular surfaces may result in early degeneration and the development of post-traumatic arthritis (Bout-Tabaku & Best 2010; Getgood & Robertson 2010).

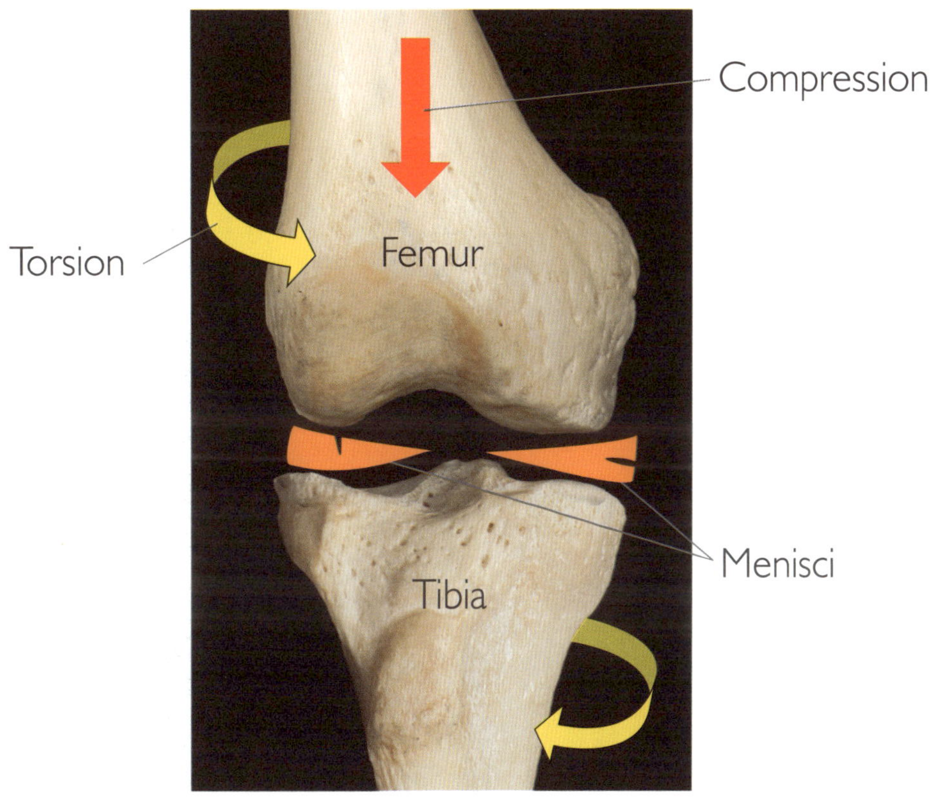

Figure 33: Meniscal tear mechanism

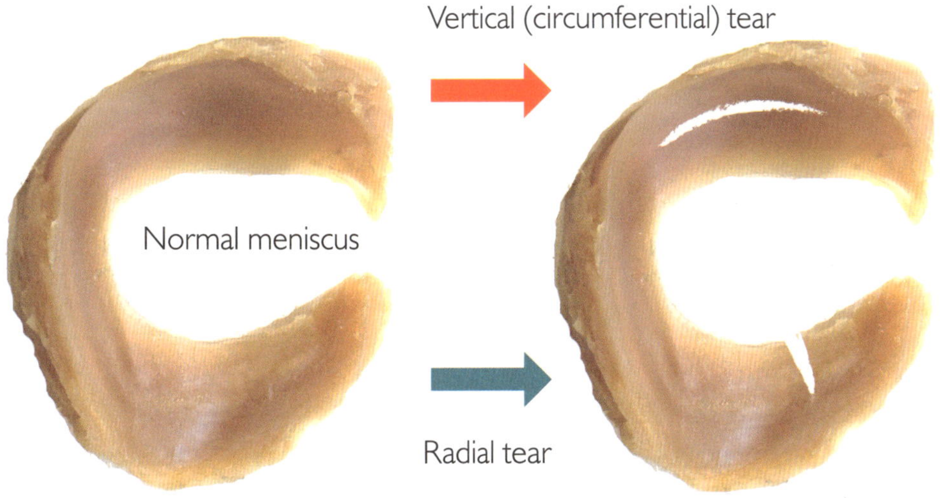

Figure 34a: There are two types of meniscal tear mechanism – vertical and radial. Circumferential vertical tears may develop into bucket-handle type tears (see Figure 34b, page 56).

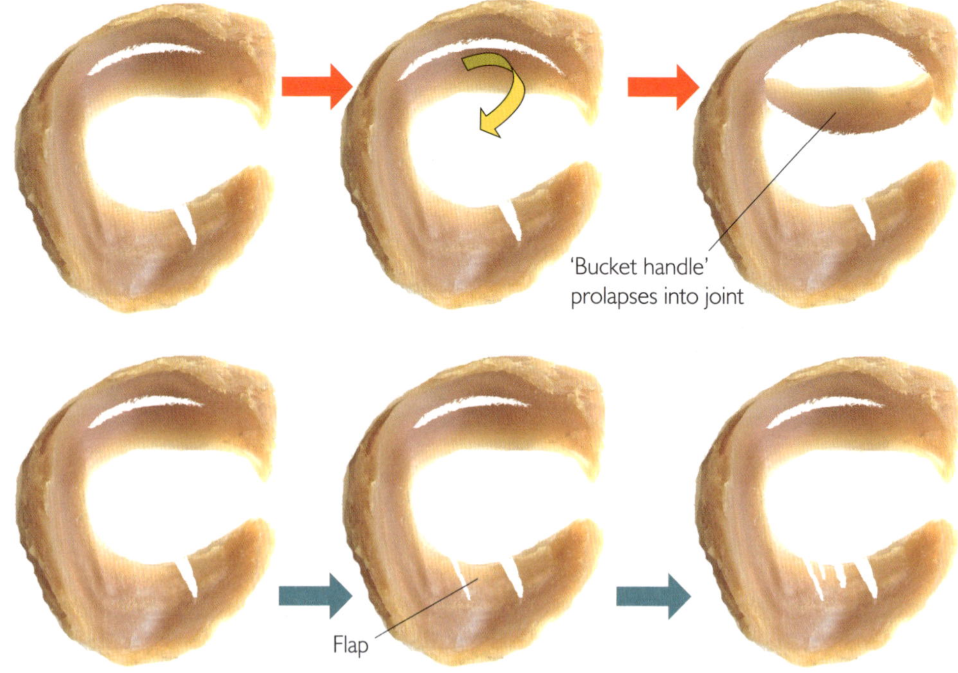

Figure 34 b: Potential development of meniscal tears

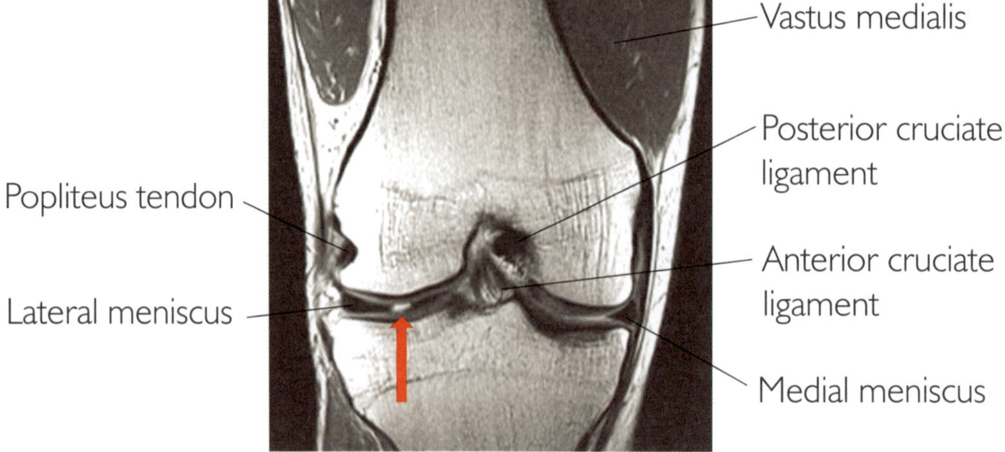

Figure 35: Coronal MRI of the knee. Note meniscal tear (arrow).

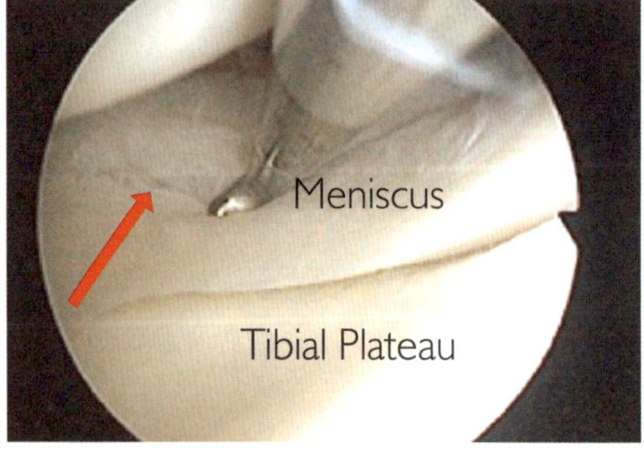

Figure 36: Arthroscopic view of a peripheral lateral vertical meniscal tear (right knee) commonly associated with ACL rupture

Problem 8

Sport – Running

Clinical history

A 35-year-old sub-elite endurance runner comes to you complaining of pain in the medial side of his left knee. He tells you that he twisted his knee while squatting three months previously. Since then he has had an intermittent sensation of something 'clicking and jamming in the knee'. He does not give any history of pre-existing knee problems.

Q1. What type of knee injury is most likely, given the mechanism and symptoms described?

Examination

Examination of his knee is unremarkable, other than a loss of terminal extension and some pain in deep flexion. He has good ligament stability and only a small effusion.

Q2. What orthopaedic manipulation tests are likely to be positive, given this presentation?

Q3. What are the usual clinical features of a meniscal tear?

Investigations

The patient tells you that his medial knee pain is having a significant effect on his ability to run and he is keen to get to the core of the problem.

Q4. What are the most appropriate imaging examinations to request and why?
What do these images (Figures P8.1a, P8.1b P8.1c) demonstrate?

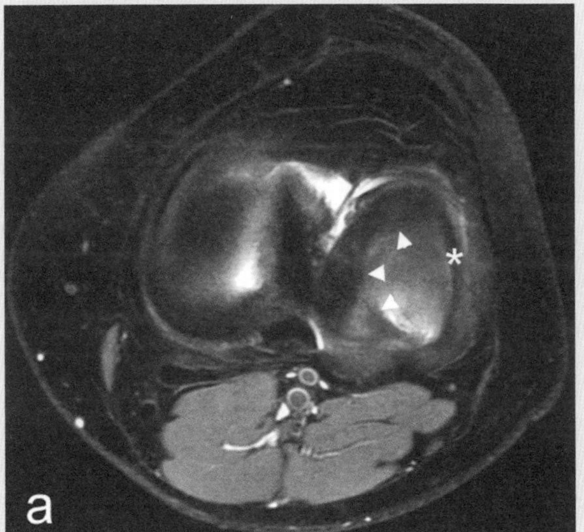

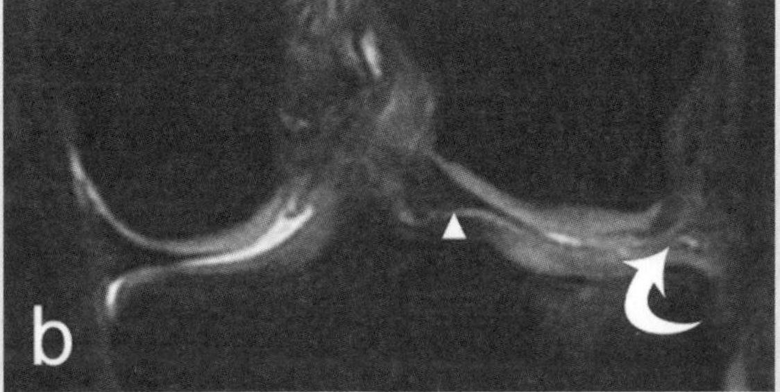

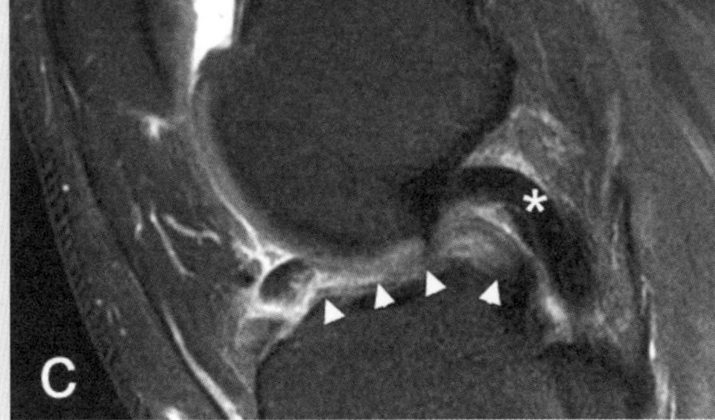

Figure P8.1a: Axial proton density sequences with fat saturation of the right knee

Figures P8.1b and P8.1c: Coronal (b) and Sagittal (c) proton density sequences with fat saturation of the right knee

Treatment

The patient is keen to know if he does have a meniscal tear whether it will need surgery to 'repair it'.

Q5. What are the key anatomical features that determine whether or not it is possible to repair a meniscal tear?

Q6. What are the positive prognostic factors regarding meniscal repair?

Problem 8: Answers

Diagnosis: Meniscal tear

A1. Medial meniscal tear. Isolated traumatic meniscal tears tend to occur as a result of loading the knee and twisting it in flexion in the younger (less than 30 years) athlete. In the older age group (over 30 years) degenerate tears can occur or become symptomatic as a result of an increase in activity such as starting to jog.

A2. a. McMurray's test.
b. Apley's test.
c. Thessaly test.

A3. a. Pain that may be localised to the joint compartment involved.
b. Mechanical symptoms of clicking or an inability to straighten the knee ('locking').
c. A feeling of instability.
d. Parameniscal cyst formation can result in localised swelling and pressure effects on local tissues (see Figure 38).

A4. An MRI, as this will confirm the diagnosis of a meniscal tear and allow an assessment of the chondral surfaces (see Figure 35, page 56). If significant degenerative changes are suspected in the knee, a plain weight-bearing x-ray may suffice.

An MRI will also determine the type of tear and allow you to assess the advisability of attempting a meniscal repair. See Figures P8.1a, P8.1b and P8.1c: (page 57) axial (a), coronal (b) and sagittal (c) proton density sequences with fat saturation of the right knee demonstrating a centrally displaced bucket handle tear of the medial meniscus. The peripheral remaining remnant of the medial meniscus is visible (asterisk a, curved arrow b). The centrally displaced fragment comprising the majority of the medial meniscus is seen within the trochlear (intercondylar) notch (arrowheads a–c). In 8.4c, the fragment closely follows the course of the PCL (asterisk), producing the 'double PCL sign'.

A5. a. Tears in the peripheral, vascular zone may be amenable to surgical repair.
b. The tear should not disrupt the circumferential collagen fibres.
c. Radial tears are generally not amenable to repair, due to the avascular nature of the central part of the meniscus, whereas vertical tears may be amenable to repair.

A6. a. Small tear
b. Peripheral
c. Young patient
d. Acute tear
e. Repair in conjunction with ligament surgery

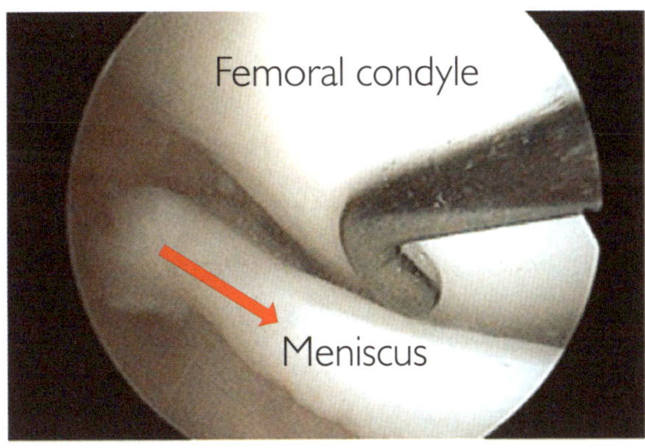

Figure 37: Arthroscopic view of a displaced 'bucket handle' tear of the lateral meniscus (left knee), causing loss of extension. Some plastic deformation has occurred.

The symptoms of meniscal tears include a gradual onset joint effusion, catching or locking of the knee with weight bearing in rotation (e.g. changing direction when running or walking) and, occasionally, locking of the knee. Common examination findings include a mild to moderate joint effusion, joint-line tenderness and a positive McMurray's test.

Meniscal cysts

Meniscal cysts (see Figure 38) can be developmental or degenerative in origin. They are often associated with a meniscal tear, especially on the lateral side. They may result from synovial fluid leaking from the main joint cavity, through the split in the meniscus, and pressing on the adjacent synovial membrane, causing it to herniate and produce a swelling.

They may be completely asymptomatic or they may present in a very similar way to meniscal tears. Occasionally they may present as a lump on the side of the knee, over the location of the meniscus.

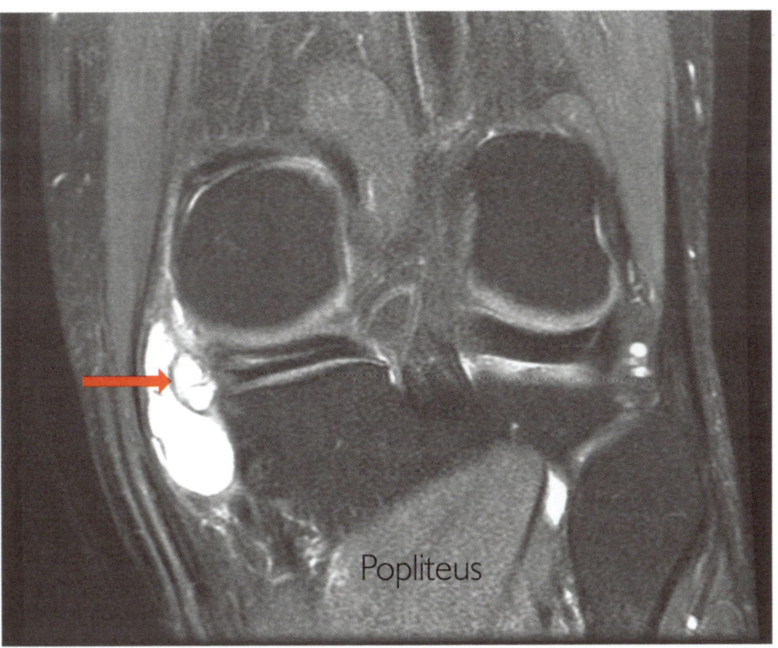

Figure 38: MRI showing a large medial meniscal cyst (red arrow) of right knee

Joint stability

Four factors are involved in stability:

1. Ligaments: These have the major role. Not only do they limit the range and direction of movement but they also hold the respective condyles together very closely. Instability is associated with ligament injuries, particularly the anterior cruciate ligament. The causes include twisting movements, jumping, falls (especially on a fully flexed knee), sudden deceleration and direct trauma. Although ligaments are frequently damaged in the knee, serious instability (such as dislocation) is uncommon.

2. Factors reinforcing the capsule: These factors supplement the action of the ligaments. They include the iliotibial band, the retinacula, and the complex insertions of muscles, particularly the semimembranosus.

3. Muscle control around the joint: This is a major factor, with co-activation of the hamstrings, quadriceps and gastrocnemius being particularly important.

4. Bony congruity: The shapes of the femoral and tibial articulating surfaces on the condyles, together with the menisci, are adapted for movement but have only a minimal role in stability. The menisci contribute to congruity to a small extent.

Ligaments

Ligaments can be classified in three groups, according to their relation to the capsule:

1. **Intra-capsular:** anterior and posterior cruciate, meniscofemoral, transverse inter-meniscal
2. **Capsular:** coronary
3. **Extra-capsular:** medial and lateral collateral, posterior oblique, oblique popliteal, popliteo-fibular

1. Intracapsular

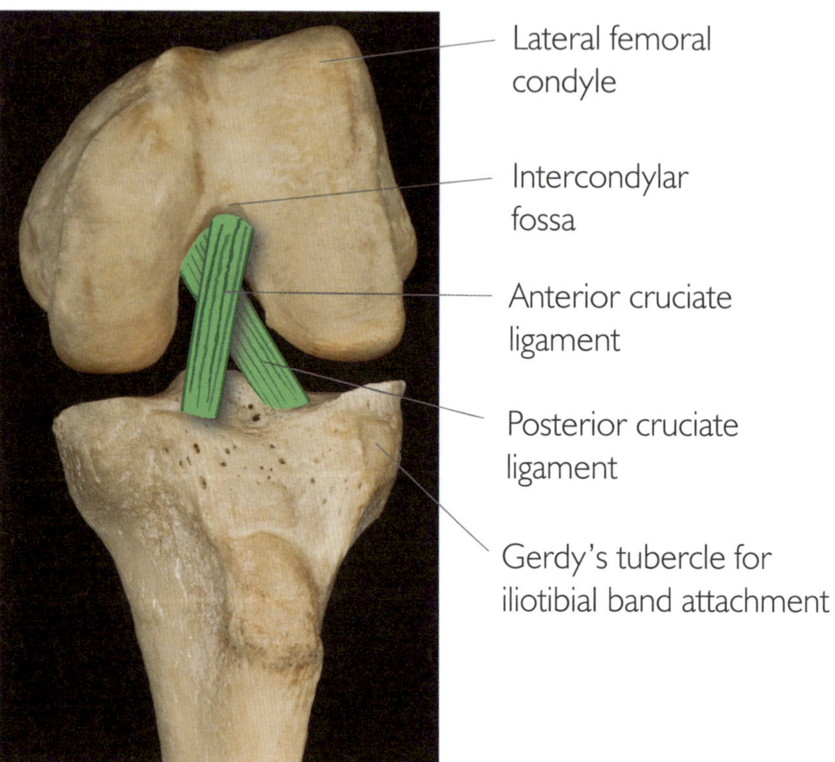

Figure 39: Frontal view of the cruciate ligaments

The cruciate ligaments

The anterior cruciate ligament (ACL) and posterior cruciate ligament (PCL) take their names from their attachment to the intercondylar eminence on the tibia. Their femoral attachments are in the intercondylar fossa of the femur (see Figure 39). The anterior ligament inclines upwards, backwards and laterally. Conversely the posterior ligament inclines upwards, forwards and medially. Although the ligaments are intra-capsular, they are covered by a sleeve of synovial membrane reflected around them from the membrane lining the posterior part of the capsule (see Figure 40. Their appearance is readily defined on MRI of the knee (see Figure 42, page 63) and also by arthroscopy (see Figures 44a and 44b, page 65).

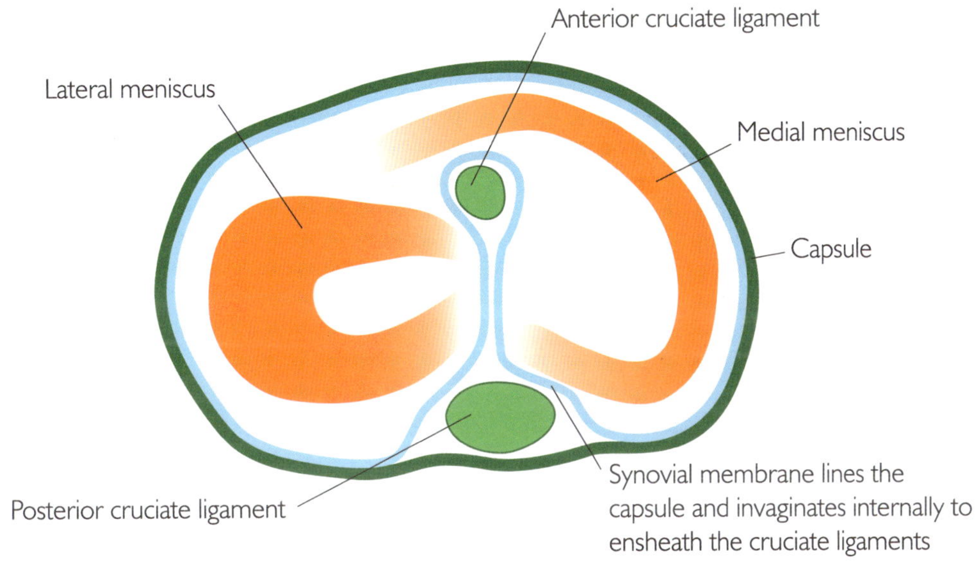

Figure 40: Menisci relationships on tibial plateau and to the cruciate ligaments and synovial membrane

The PCL is *significantly thicker* than the ACL (see Figure 29, page 52). Given its smaller size and role in resisting antero-lateral tibial rotation, it is not surprising that a large proportion (80%) of cruciate ligament injuries involve the anterior ligament. Stretching or tearing of these ligaments causes instability of the knee and may result from twisting, falling, jumping, sudden deceleration or direct trauma. They are commonly injured in football (see Figure 45, page 65). The posterior ligament is particularly vulnerable to falling on a flexed knee.

Actions of the PCL and ACL

The PCL has a prime role in knee stability. It resists forward displacement of the femur on the tibia, as when walking down stairs. It also resists posterior displacement of the tibia. Throughout flexion and extension, it remains taut by virtue of having two components: a larger antero-lateral part, which is tight during flexion; and a smaller posteromedial part, which is tight during extension.

The ACL resists posterior displacement of the femur or antero-lateral displacement of the tibia and hyperextension.

The movements in a sagittal plane resisted by these ligaments are shown in Figure 41, and damage to them is shown in Figures 43 and 44b (pages 64,65).

ACL and PCL both also resist torsion. Complete rupture of the ACL results in an antero-lateral rotatory instability.

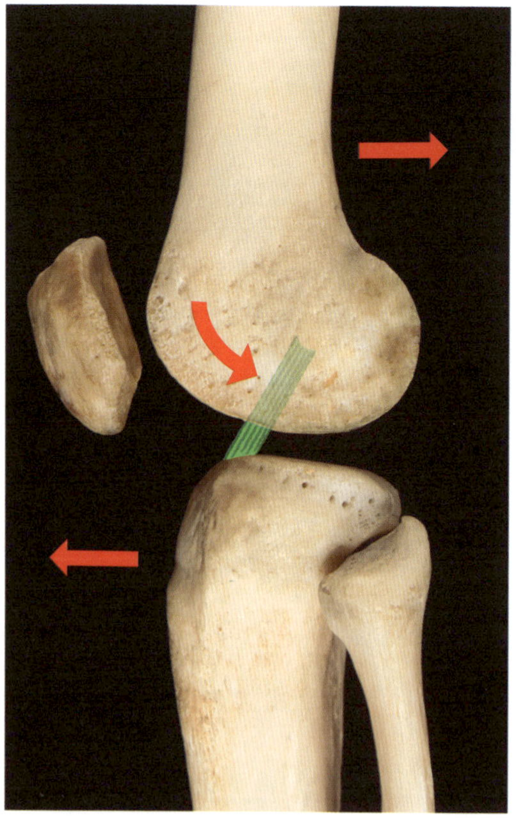

Figure 41: Arrangement of cruciate ligaments and mechanism of tears: anterior cruciate ligament

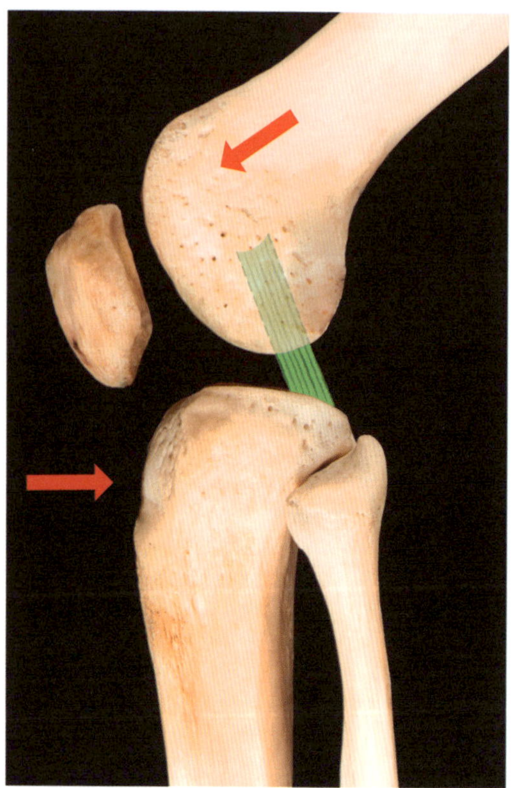

Figure 42: Arrangement of cruciate ligaments and mechanism of tears: posterior cruciate ligament. Arrows indicate the direction of displacement of bones.

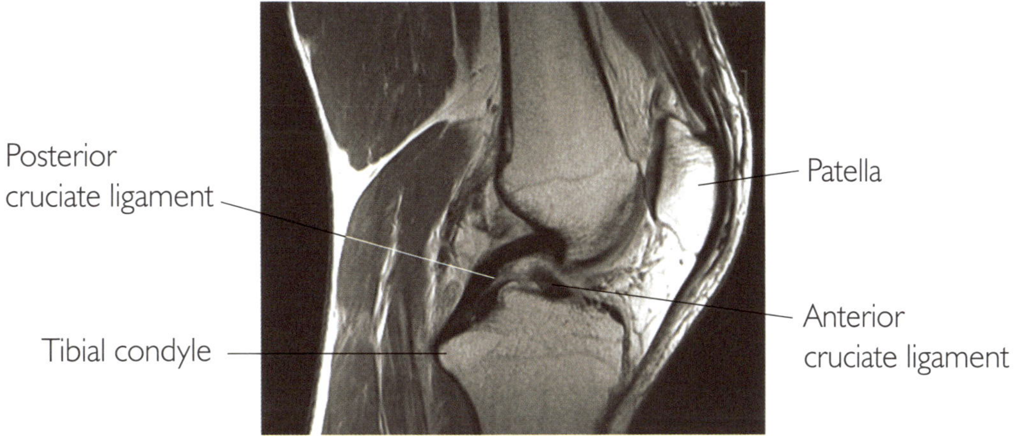

Figure 43: Sagittal MRI of knee showing normal cruciate ligaments. Note the difference in thickness of ligaments. Compare with Figure 29.

Problem 9

Sport – Rugby

Clinical history

A 40-year-old rugby player presents to the clinic complaining of progressive anterior and medial knee pain, particularly with prolonged sitting and descending stairs. He does not describe any memorable injury but has had 'a number of knocks over the years'. He gets a crunching sensation on squatting but no true locking. He does not describe any symptoms of instability such as 'giving way' of the knee.

Q1. What is the most likely diagnosis?

Examination

Examination of the patient reveals a small knee joint effusion. There is medial joint-line tenderness on palpation and a small amount of patellofemoral crepitus on active knee flexion and extension, and passive medial and lateral gliding of the patella. Ligament testing reveals moderate laxity with a positive posterior drawer test. Anterior drawer testing and Lachman's testing are symmetrical with the opposite knee.

Q2. What is your clinical diagnosis?

Q3. Why are clinical features of patellofemoral and medial compartment pathology both present?

Investigations

In view of the patient's ongoing symptoms, an MRI scan is obtained (see Figure 43).

Q4. What is the observed abnormality?

Treatment

The patient has seen his doctor who has prescribed him non-steroidal anti-inflammatory medication.

Q5. What treatment options are available?

Q6. Are any of these treatment options likely to alter the natural history of the condition?

Problem 9: Answers

Diagnosis: Chronic posterior cruciate ligament (PCL) rupture with associated patellofemoral osteoarthritis

A1. 1. Patellofemoral pathology (Arthritis/Osteochondral injury).
2. Posterior horn medial meniscal tear/cyst.
3. Chronic posterior cruciate ligament (PCL) rupture.

A2. Chronic PCL disruption.

A3. In the chronically PCL deficient knee, altered biomechanics result in increased patellofemoral loading and increased antero-posterior movement in the medial compartment. This leads to medial meniscal and chondral pathology in chronic cases.

A4. The MRI scan demonstrates signal change representing disruption of the PCL, along with mild chondral cartilage degradation of the medial femoral condyle and patellofemoral joint with some underlying bone oedema.

A5. 1. Non-surgical options include modification of activities, functional bracing and a knee muscle strengthening and control programme.
2. Surgical approaches range from treating chondral or meniscal pathology arthroscopically to osteotomies or ligament reconstruction in an attempt to alter the biomechanics of the knee.

A6. The available evidence is conflicting regarding the likelihood of changing the long-term prognosis with surgical intervention. Complete resolution of symptoms is unlikely.

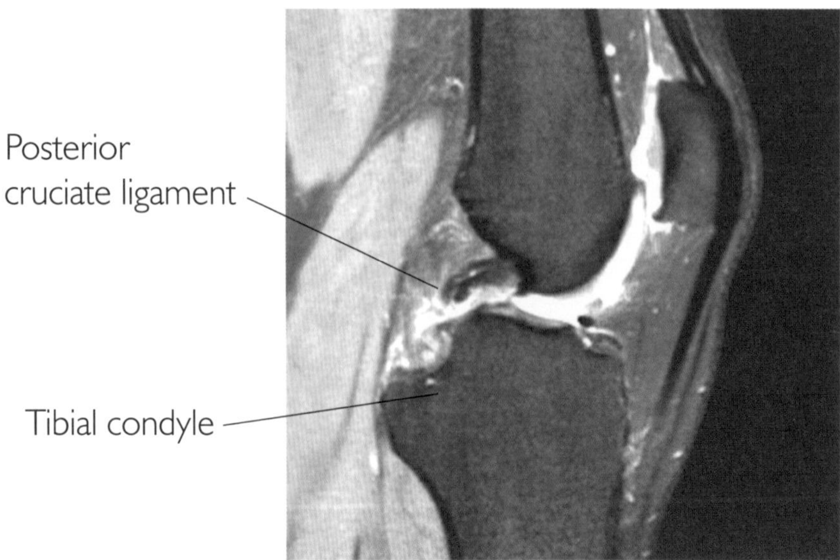

Figure 44. Sagittal MRI of the knee showing ruptured posterior cruciate ligament

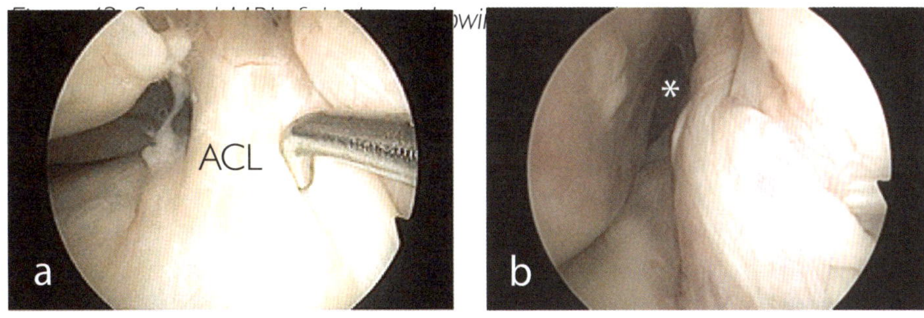

Figure 45

a: Arthroscopic view of a normal anterior cruciate ligament running from infero-medial to posterolateral in the femoral notch (right knee)

b: Ruptured anterior cruciate ligament (right knee) with 'empty lateral wall sign' (shown by asterisk)

Problem 10

Sport – Football (Soccer)

Clinical history

A 24-year-old local league football player was trying to avoid an opponent when his studs 'caught in the turf'. He recalls a 'cracking' sound from his left knee, with immediate pain as he fell to the ground. Despite his best attempts he was unable to resume play and had to be helped from the field. He was initially able to bear weight but within two to three hours his knee became swollen and remained so for the next few days. He attended the emergency department the following day, where x-rays were performed.

Q1. What are the most likely diagnoses?

Examination

Examination one week after the injury reveals a moderate to large knee joint effusion. The collateral ligaments do not show any evidence of laxity and the patient is able to perform a straight leg raise with discomfort. The patient has difficulty fully flexing the knee, due to a feeling of tightness in the back of the knee.

Q2. What clinical findings would suggest an injury to the anterior cruciate ligament?

Q3. What type of instability does an isolated anterior cruciate ligament injury result in and why?

Investigations

The x-rays taken were reported as 'no abnormality detected'.

Q4. What are the next most appropriate forms of examination?

Treatment

The athlete tells you that he is keen to return to playing the same level of football once or twice per week.

Q5. What should his initial treatment consist of?

Q6. What needs to be considered in determining whether or not to perform surgical reconstruction?

Problem 10: Answers

Diagnosis: Anterior cruciate ligament (ACL) injury

A1. a. ACL rupture.
b. Patellar dislocation.
c. Acute meniscal tear (unlikely).

A2. a. A moderate to large effusion.
b. A positive Lachman's test.
c. A positive anterior drawer test.
d. Apprehension when asked to change direction of gait.

A3. An isolated ACL injury will result in an antero-lateral rotatory instability. This is due to the orientation of the ligament, which provides both antero-posterior and rotatory support to the knee joint.

A4. An MRI scan and arthroscopy (see Figures 44a and 44b) would be helpful to confirm the likely clinical diagnosis and to assess the knee for additional common injuries such as lateral meniscal tears (in particular, the posterior horn, which is 'pinched' during the injury), bone bruising, chondral injuries and any associated ligament injuries.

A5. a. This would be determined by the pattern of injury but should include application of the POLICE regimen in the initial phase.
b. As the inflammatory process diminishes, treatment goals should include physical therapy and exercise rehabilitation aimed at restoring a full range of movement of the knee and then optimising knee flexor, extensor and synergist muscle strength and control. Return to sport can be considered if the player is able to progress to end-stage rehabilitation, including high-load, multi-directional, football-specific activities without significant pain, swelling or 'giving way' of the knee.

A6. a. The degree and frequency of functional instability (i.e. 'giving way') experienced by the patient.
b. The patient's long-term sporting, occupational and recreational goals.
c. The patient's general health status.
d. The timing of any reconstructive procedure would depend on the pattern of injury, as well as social, occupational and sporting factors.

Meniscofemoral ligament

This ligament is attached to the posterior border of the lateral meniscus (see Figure 29, page 52) and becomes closely associated with the posterior cruciate ligament as it passes upward and forward to its attachment on the lateral side of the medial femoral condyle in the intercondylar fossa (see Figure 46). It may pass anterior or posterior to the cruciate ligament to reach its attachment. The ligament plays an essential role in holding the meniscus in close contact with the inferior surface of the lateral condyle during flexion and extension of the joint.

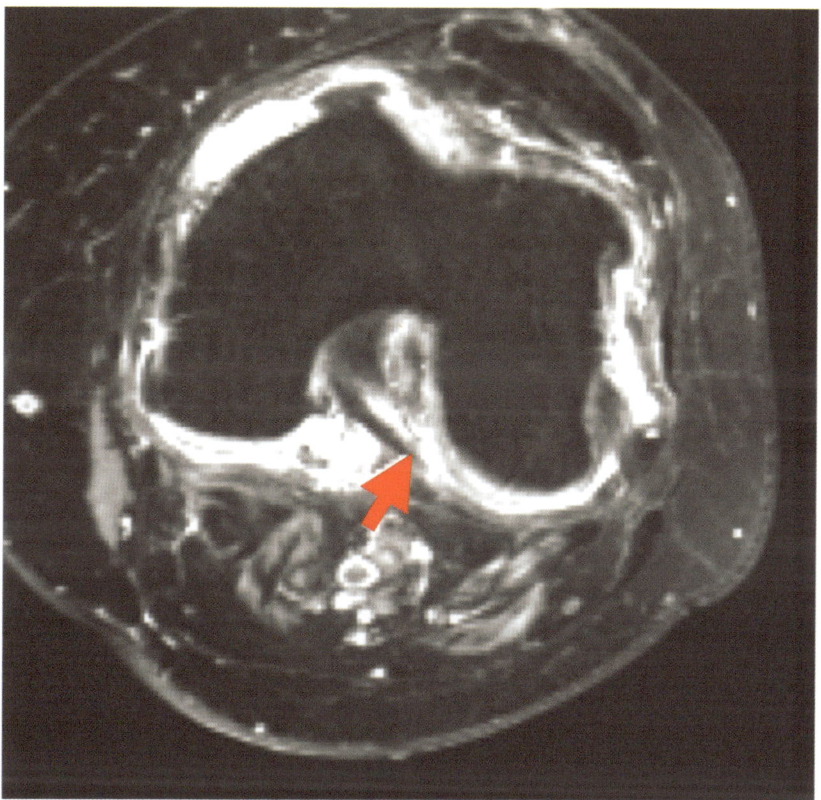

Figure 46: Coronal MRI of the knee showing the meniscofemoral ligament (red arrow)

Transverse ligament

This short ligament lies just deep to the anterior part of the capsule and close to the tibial plateau. It connects the anterior horn of the medial meniscus with the anterior border of the lateral meniscus.

10

Extra-articular ligaments and corner complexes

Capsular ligaments

The coronary ligaments are essentially deeper parts of the capsule, which are attached to the outer margins of the menisci and to the subjacent margins of the tibial articular cartilage and bony condyles (see Figure 47).

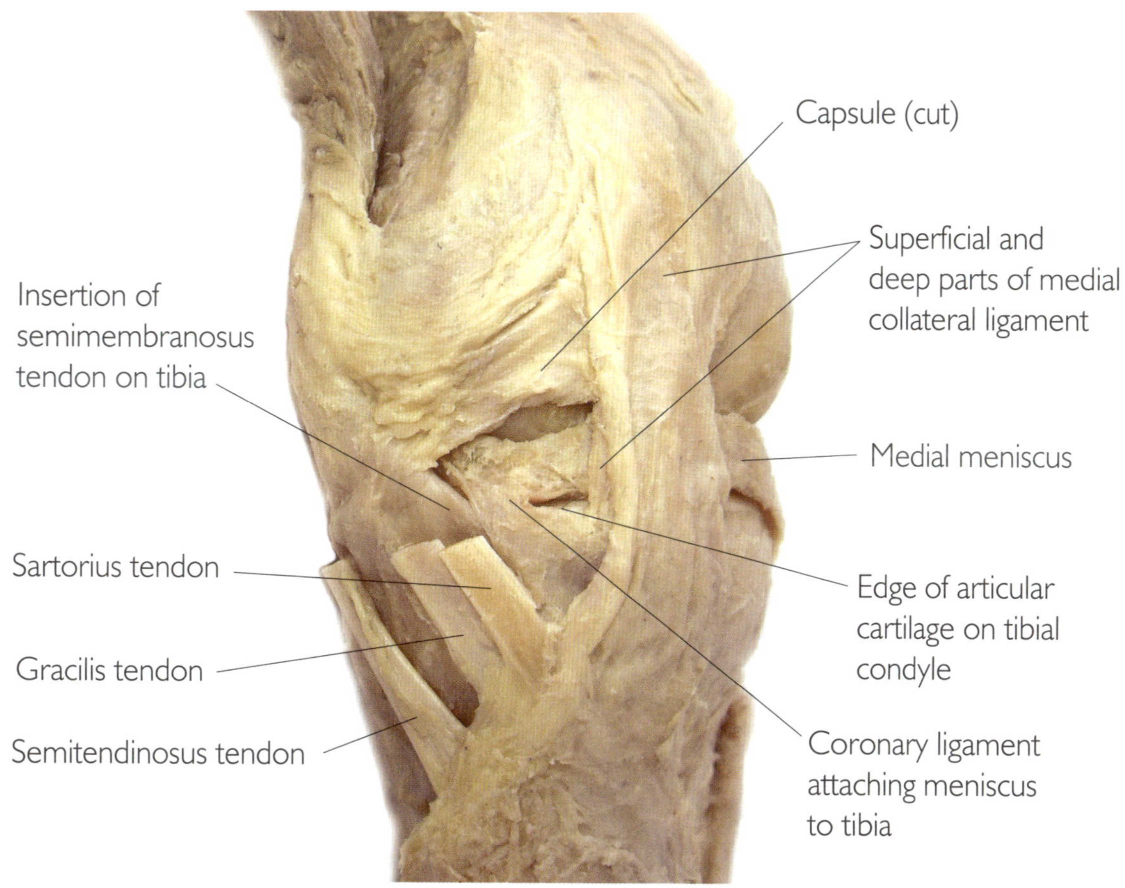

Figure 47: Structures forming posteromedial corner complex. Note: medial collateral and coronary ligaments.

Extra-capsular ligaments

Collateral ligaments

The collateral ligaments are located on each side of the joint capsule (see Figures 28, 29 and 30, pages 51,52 and 53). The lateral ligament is a well-defined cord-like structure (see Figure 29). It is attached proximally to the lateral femoral epicondyle and distally to the head of the fibula, close to its apex. The medial ligament is much broader and less well-defined (see Figure 47, page 69), tending to fuse with the capsule. Proximally it is attached to the medial femoral epicondyle. Distally it broadens considerably, with a deep part attaching close to the edge of the articular surface of the medial tibial condyle and to the medial meniscus. A superficial part attaches to the more distal part of the tibial condyle and often extends down to the upper part of the tibial shaft.

Action: The two ligaments together become taut on full extension of the knee, preventing hyperextension (see Figure 48). With the knee extended, they give lateral (side-to-side) stability.

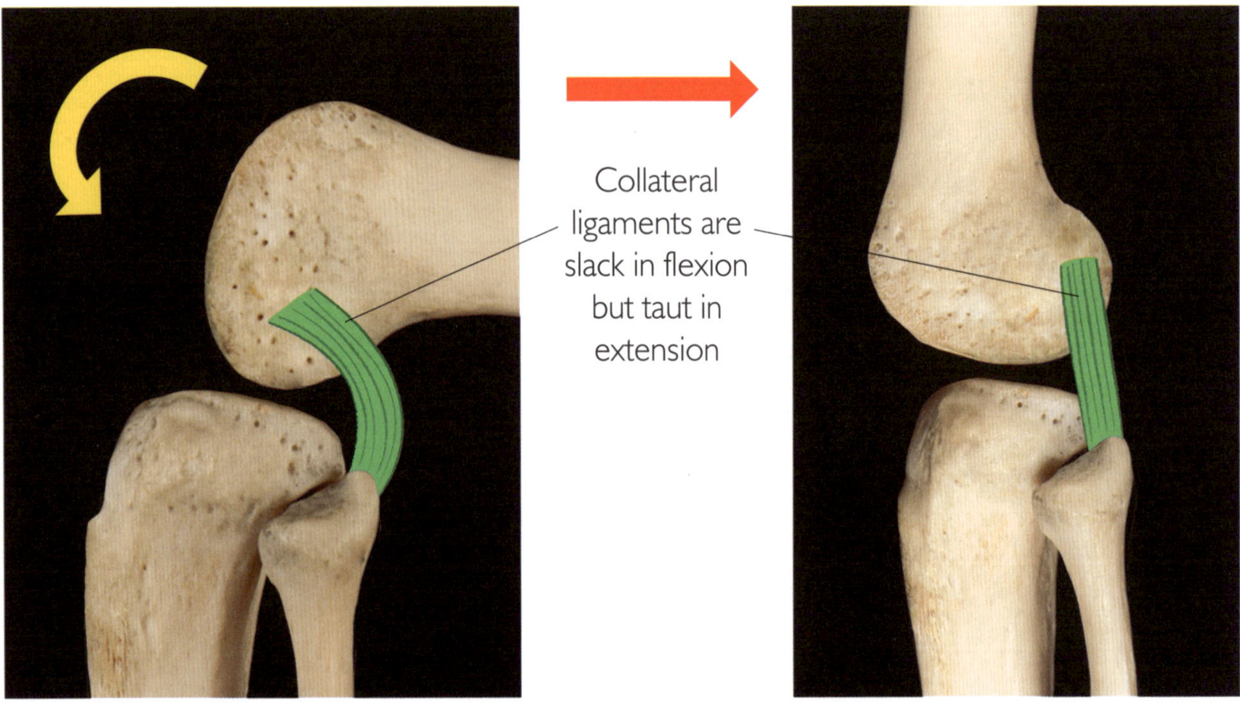

Figure 48: Effect of flexion and extension on collateral ligaments of the knee

Problem 11

Sport – Tobogganing

Clinical history

A 45-year-old man was tobogganing with his family when his left foot caught in the snow as he tried to stop himself. He felt a sharp pain as his knee was forced into a valgus position. He said he felt a tearing sensation and had significant pain on weight bearing.

Q1. What are the differential diagnoses?

Examination

On examination three days later, there was no evidence of effusion, or any knee ligament instability, but valgus stress testing was markedly painful.

Q2. Given this finding, where should attention be particularly focused during the examination that will help to identify the likely injury and its severity?

Investigations

An MRI of the knee is thought to be the most relevant investigation.

Q3. What is demonstrated in the area indicated by the white arrow? (see Figure P11.1, below)

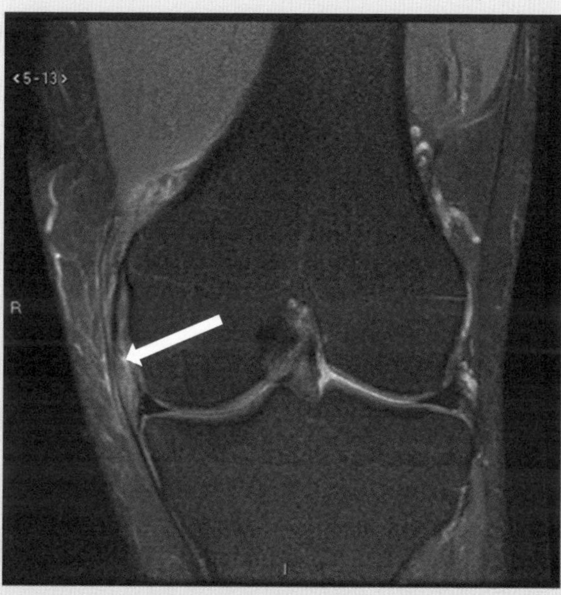

Figure P11.1: Coronal knee MRI

Treatment

Q4. What treatment options are available?

Problem 11: Answers

Diagnosis: Medial collateral ligament (MCL) injury

A1. MCL injury. Medial meniscal tear.

A2. The key factor is to identify the area of maximal tenderness and palpate the whole length of the medial collateral ligament. Avulsions/tears often occur at either the proximal or distal ends. Joint-line tenderness may imply a meniscal injury.

The structural integrity of the MCL and supporting structures should be assessed in full extension and slight flexion. Injury can be graded as:

- **I** a sprain (minimal structural damage)
- **II** a tear (with some residual structural integrity)
- **III** a significant tear (with loss of structural integrity)

In the case of a grade II or III sprain, it is important to rule out injury to the ACL, which is a secondary restraint to valgus loading.

A3. Increased signal around the MCL. Fibres intact. Suggests a high-grade sprain.

A4. The majority of MCL injuries can be treated conservatively. In the initial phase, analgesia, splinting (two to four weeks at 30° for optimal ligament alignment), and a POLICE regimen can control symptoms. This should generally be followed by a period of bracing, to allow the ligament to heal without exposure to excessive valgus forces. Surgical reconstruction of the medial collateral ligament is rarely required in the absence of an associated ACL injury.

Oblique popliteal ligament

This ligament is part of the triple attachment of the semimembranosus tendon in the region of the knee. It forms a distinct thickening in the posterior part of the capsule, passing from the principal insertion in the groove on the posteromedial side of the medial tibial condyle, upwards and laterally towards the upper border of the lateral femoral condyle (see Figures 16a, 49 and 56, pages 33,72,77).

Action: The ligament becomes taut as the knee is extended and is part of the ligamentous mechanism, preventing over-extension.

Posterior oblique ligament

This ligament is formed by an extension from the medial collateral ligament onto the posteromedial part of the capsule and close to the insertion of the semimembranosus tendon (see Figures 49 and 57a, page 78). It is tensed by stretching of the collateral ligament.

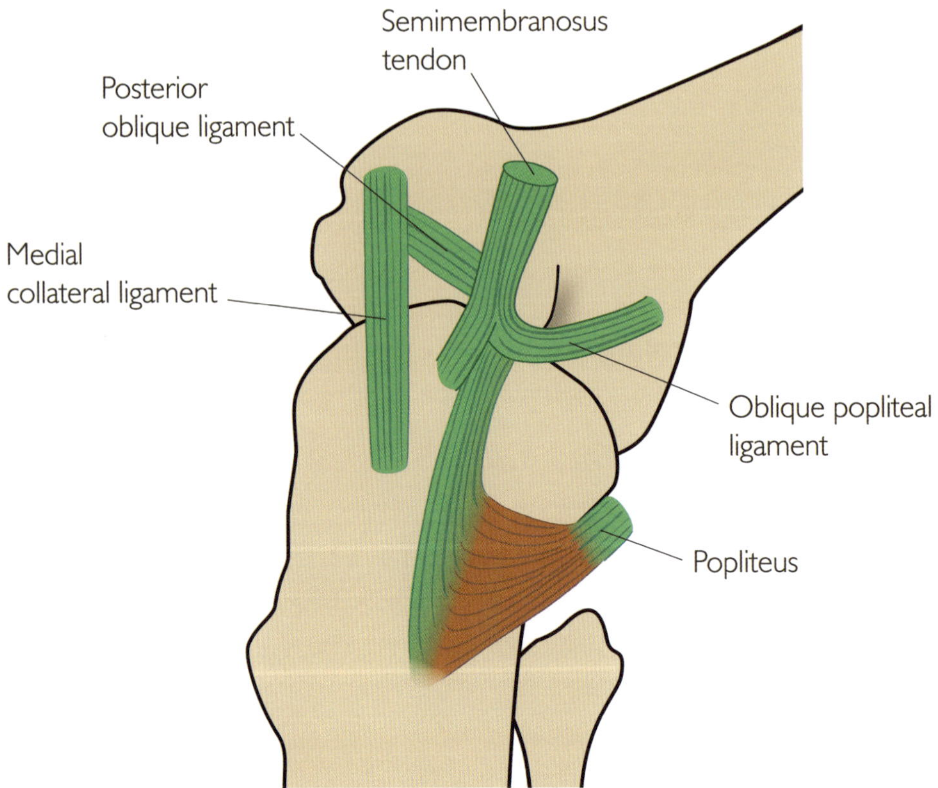

Figure 49: Medial collateral and the two oblique ligaments

The stabilising functions of ligaments

These are:

- Antero-posterior stability (cruciate ligaments)
- Side-to-side stability and resisting varus and valgus stresses (collateral ligaments)
- Preventing hyperextension (anterior cruciate, medial and lateral collateral ligaments, oblique popliteal and posterior oblique ligaments)

All the ligaments that prevent hyperextension fulfil *two fundamental roles:*

1. They help to maintain a completely upright posture. When standing fully upright, body weight lies in front of the transverse axis of the knee joint and this tends to over-extend the knee. This is countered by those ligaments that prevent over-extension (see below).

2. They control knee movements.

The knee is a modified hinge joint. Its principal movements are flexion by hamstring muscles and extension by quadriceps femoris. The movements occur over a range of about 135°. During the process of extension, the femoral condyles undergo a combination of hinge, gliding and pivot movements in relation to the tibial plateau. As the knee moves towards full extension, the femur (together with the lateral meniscus) rotates medially on the tibia. This movement has been termed the 'screw-home mechanism' and it is governed by the position of the taut anterior cruciate ligament.

The posterior cruciate ligament also becomes taut as full extension is reached. At this point, the various ligaments (collateral, anterior cruciate and oblique popliteal) that limit extension become taut, preventing any further extension. In this position, the joint is described as 'locked'. This might be interpreted to mean that the joint has become 'fixed' in position and cannot be moved but this is not so, since the joint is free to move into flexion. It should not be confused with pathological locking. When initiating flexion, the femur is rotated laterally by the action of the popliteus muscle.

Supplementary factors assisting stability of the knee joint

In addition to the capsule itself and the collateral ligaments, a number of adjacent structures (particularly tendons inserting close to the joint) strengthen the knee and help to maintain its stability. These are particularly related to the posterolateral and posteromedial sides (corners). If these structures are injured, the adjacent capsule may be damaged and this will result in instability.

The posterolateral complex

There are a number of structures on the posterolateral side of the knee that contribute to the stability of this part of the joint and reinforce the capsule. They can be considered as three layers, with the capsule contributing to the deepest layer (see Figure 50). They include the iliotibial tract (see Figure 51), biceps femoris tendon, the patellar retinaculum, the popliteus tendon and arcuate ligament, popliteo-fibular ligament and fabello-fibular ligament.

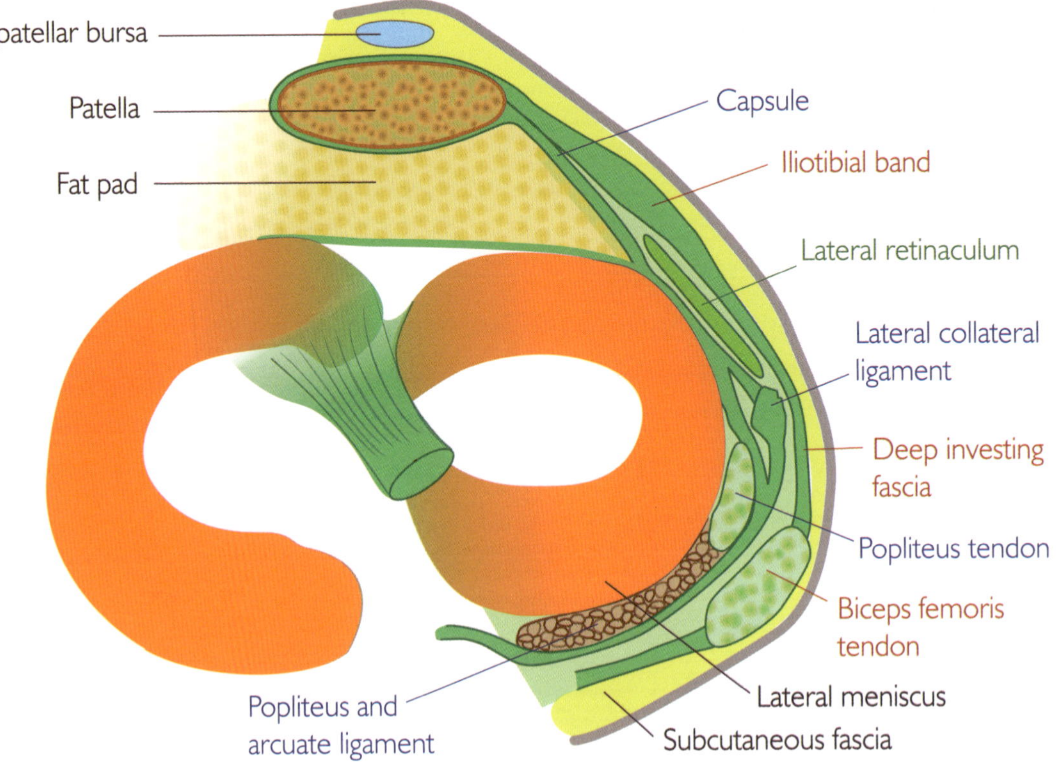

Figure 50: The posterolateral complex.
Key to layers in complex: Layer 1 = red, Layer 2 = green, Layer 3 = blue.

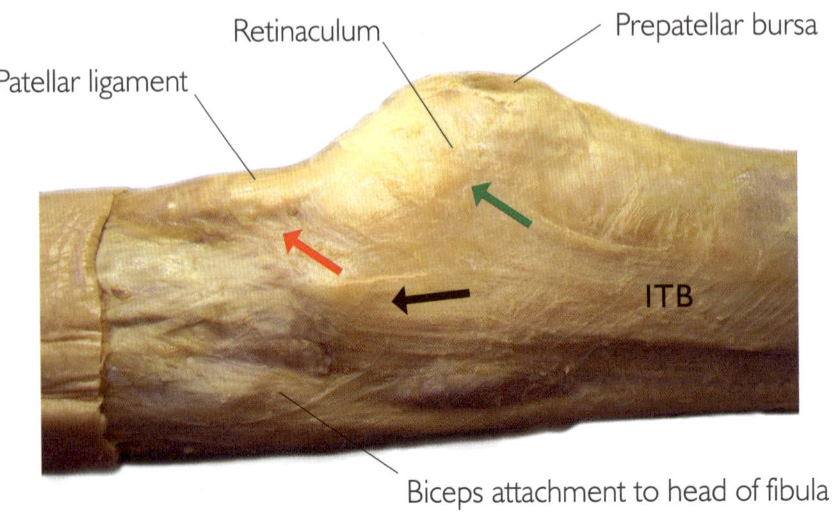

Figure 51: The iliotibial band (ITB) reinforces the lateral side of the capsule

The green arrow shows fibres in the region of the lateral retinaculum, the black arrow the fibres passing to the main attachment on the tibia. The red arrow shows fibres passing anterior to the patellar ligament. They are well developed and pass across the front of the ligament to be continuous with those on the opposite side. Their location and size suggest that they stabilise the patellar ligament and prevent bow-stringing during knee extension.

The popliteus muscle lies deeply in the lowest part of the floor of the popliteal fossa and arises from the proximal part of the posterior surface of the tibia, above the soleal line. Its tendon passes upward and laterally towards the lateral condyle of the femur, which it approaches from within the capsule of the knee joint (see Figures 52 and 53). It has a triple attachment. As it pierces the capsule, some of its fibres attach to the capsule.

Within the joint, the tendon is ensheathed by synovial membrane and some of the fibres attach to the lateral meniscus. Continuing towards the condyle, the tendon separates the lateral border of the meniscus from the lateral collateral ligament and then attaches to a groove on the side of the condyle, below the epicondyle and within the joint. The popliteus medially rotates the tibia during terminal knee extension. Cumulative tibial external rotation stress, as seen in bend runners and downhill walkers, may induce popliteus tendinopathy. Symptoms are pain at the back of the knee or on the posterolateral side, where there may also be tenderness over the condyle. Medial rotation of the leg, especially against resistance, produces pain.

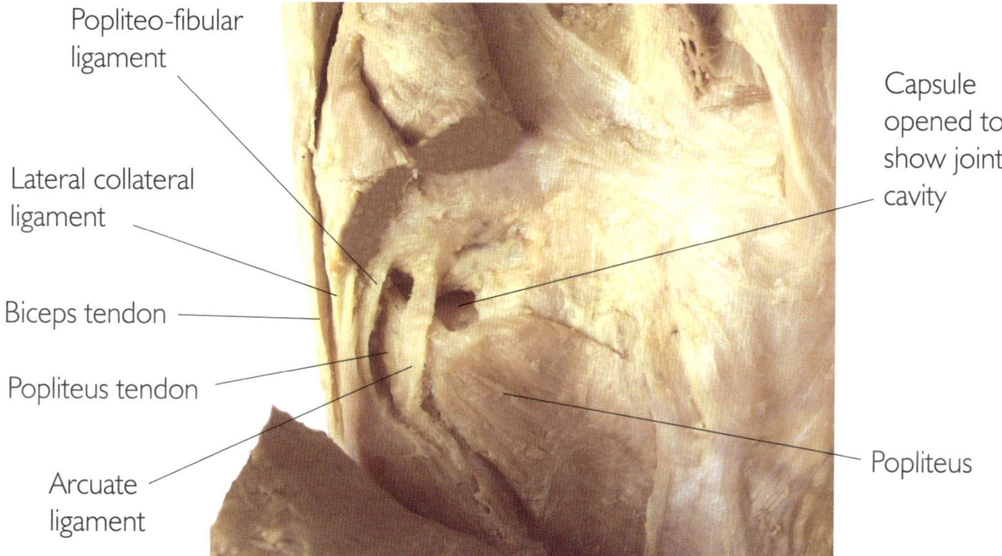

Figure 52: Popliteus muscle and tendon

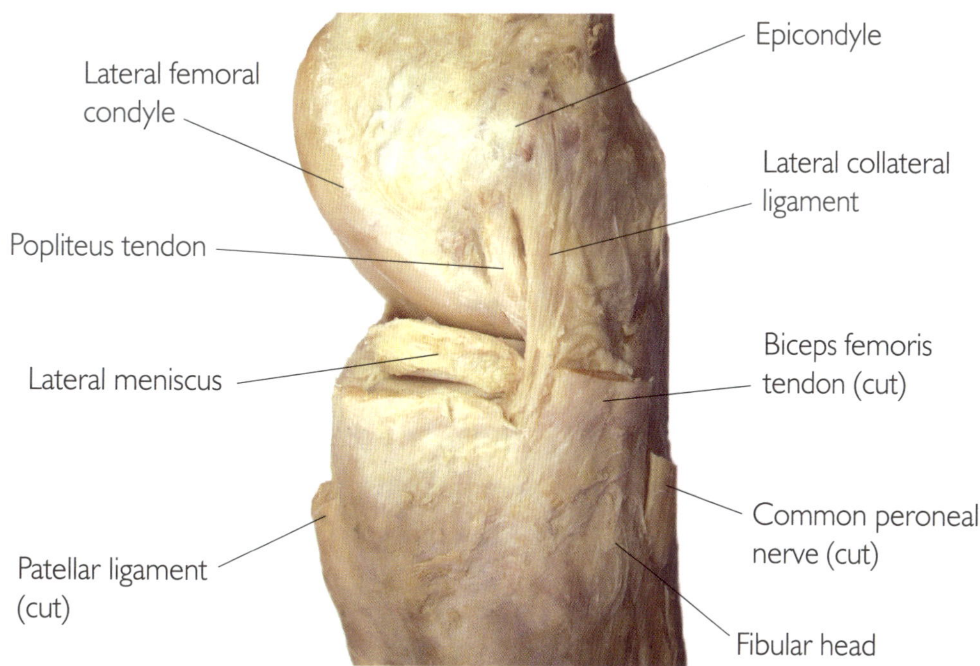

Figure 53: Popliteus tendon attachment on lateral femoral condyle. The joint capsule has been removed.

The posteromedial complex

Components strengthening the medial side of the knee joint can be classified in three groups according to their location around the circumference of this part of the joint. In the anterior third is the medial retinaculum; in the middle third are the superficial and deep parts of the medial collateral ligament; whilst in the posterior third there are several tendons, including sartorius, gracilis and semitendinosus, combining to form the extensive pes anserina, attaching to the tibia. Also in the posterior third is a major structure, the semimembranosus. These structures in the posterior third make up the posteromedial complex (see Figure 54).

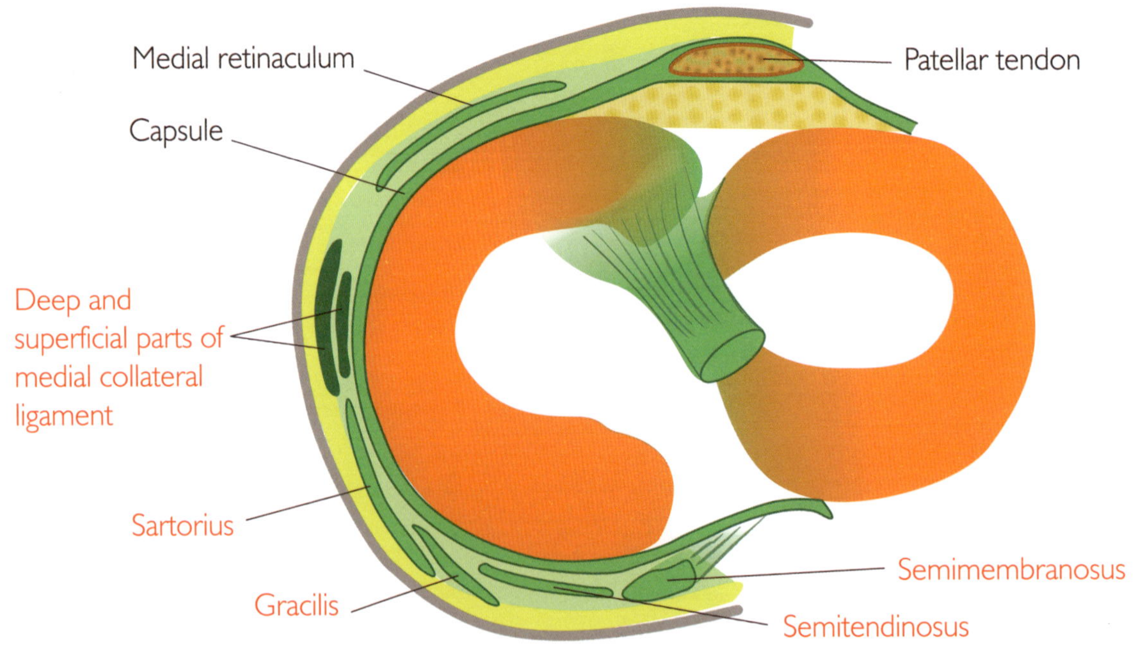

Figure 54: The posteromedial complex
The structures contributing to the posteromedial corner are labelled in red

The major factor in this complex is focused around the semimembranosus tendon as it passes to its principal attachment on the medial condyle of the tibia, together with several extensions from the tendon (see Figures 54, 55 and 56). Acting with the tendon, these extensions help to reinforce the capsule and stabilise the posteromedial side of the joint.

There are three categories of injury, which may occur concurrently:

1. Tearing of the semimembranosus tendon
2. Tearing in the region of the posterior oblique ligament (see Figure 57, page 78)
3. Tearing of the capsule from the periphery of the medial meniscus.

Injuries to the nearby medial collateral ligament may also involve the semimembranosus extensions.

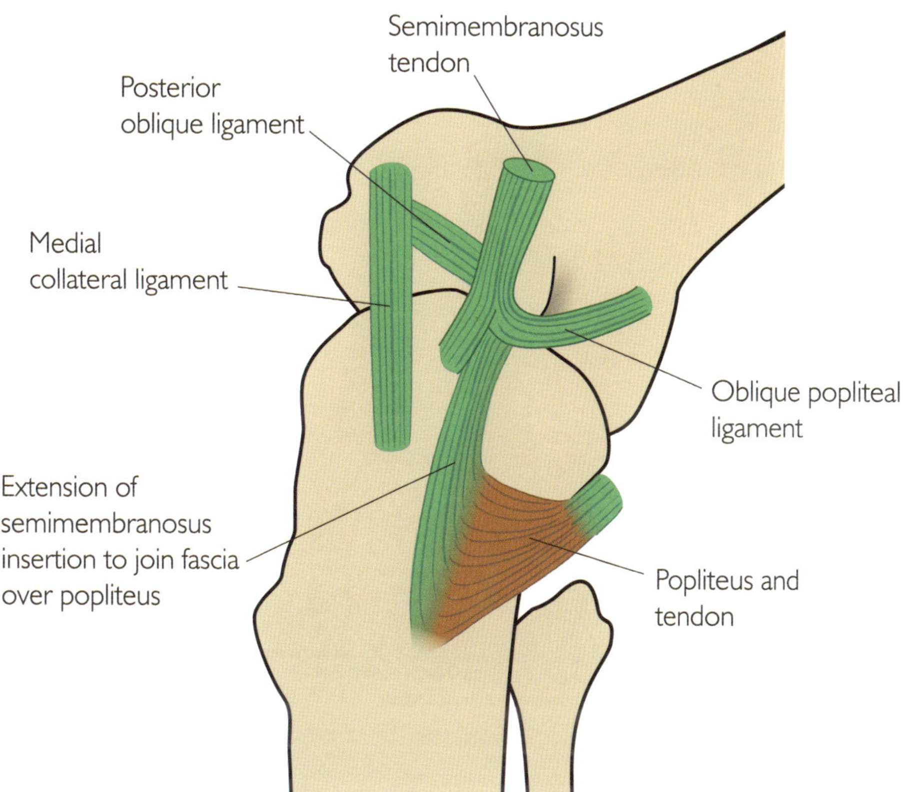

Figure 55: Extensions of semimembranosus insertion and adjacent ligaments

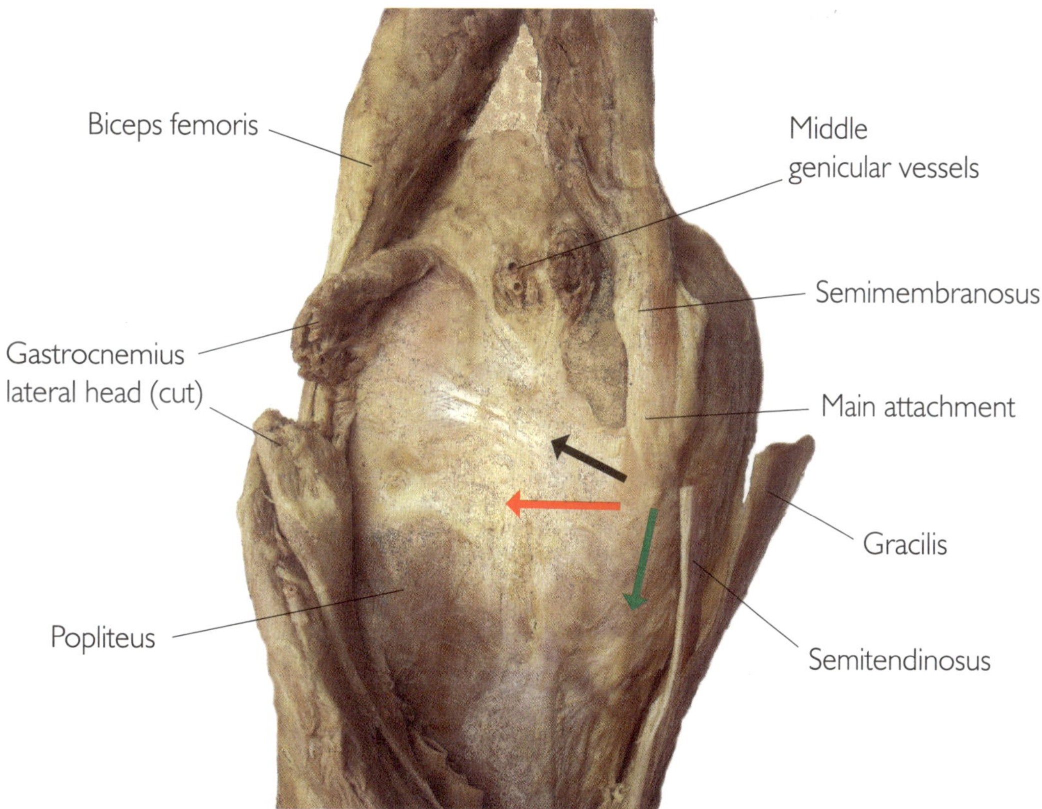

Figure 56: The posteromedial complex. Main insertions of semimembranosus tendon. Black arrow – posterior oblique popliteal ligament, red arrow – arcuate ligament, green arrow – extension fusing with popliteus fascia.

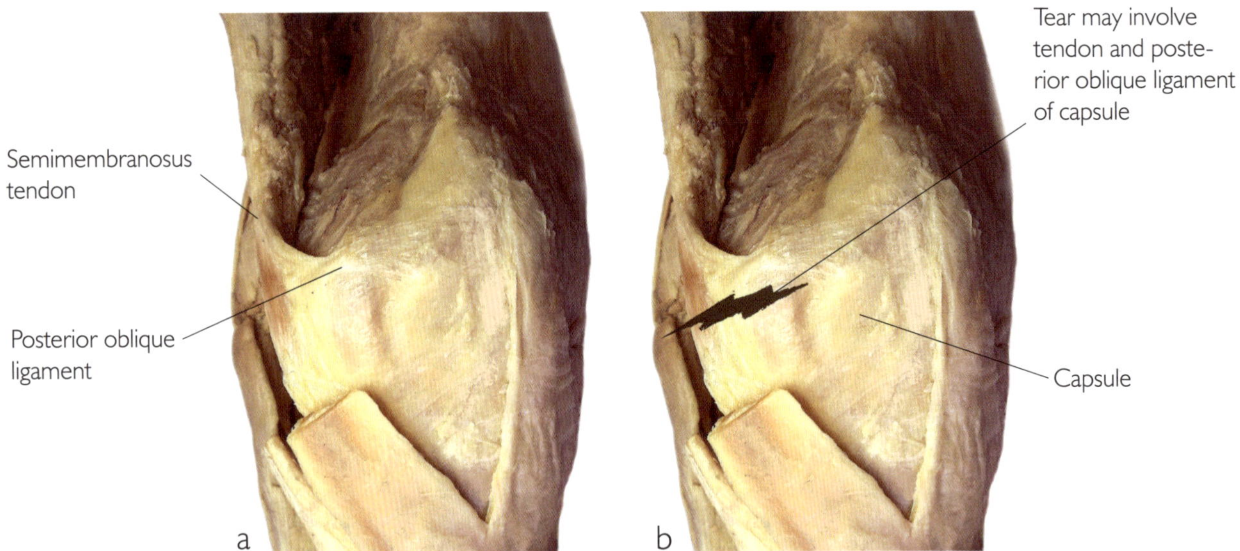

Figure 57 a: Semimembranosus tendon and posterior oblique ligament
b: Tear of semimembranosus tendon and posterior oblique ligament

Knee joint dislocation

Knee joint dislocation is uncommon, usually occurring as a result of motor vehicle accidents or during high-force or high-velocity sports. The most frequent forms are *anterior*, which accounts for about 40% and is usually caused by extreme hyperextension of the joint, and *posterior*, accounting for about 33%. Extra-articular structures that are particularly vulnerable to damage include the popliteal artery and vein, which threaten viability of the leg and foot and common peroneal nerve. The ligamentous pattern of injury depends on the mechanism of injury and involves various combinations of ligament injury, the most common being ACL, PCL and MCL (Robertson, Nutton & Keating 2006).

Problem 12

Sport – Skiing

Clinical history

A 45-year-old businessman was skiing off-piste when his left ski ran into a tree stump under the snow. His bindings failed to release. He felt immediate pain and felt the knee 'pop'. He remembers the leg lying at an odd angle. He was unable to ski on and has been brought into the medical facility on an extraction stretcher. His left knee is in a splint. His boots have been removed.

Q1. Apart from bony injury what main structures might have been damaged?

Q2. What are the important things to assess initially?

Examination

Examination of the knee reveals marked swelling of the joint. The overall alignment is good. On lifting the foot to remove the patient's clothing, the knee falls into recurvatum and external rotation.

Q3. What is the most likely diagnosis?

The physical examination is limited by pain.

Q4. What examination findings might alert you to a serious ligament injury?

Investigations

There is some discussion among the medical staff regarding the appropriateness of obtaining an x-ray of the knee.

Q5. What would be the advantages and disadvantages of an x-ray of the knee in this situation?

Treatment

You are asked to decide how best to manage the patient.

Q6. What should you do in the immediate term?

Q7. What treatment may be required in the longer term?

Problem 12: Answers

Diagnosis: Multi-ligament injury

A1. The joint capsule.
Ligaments – collateral, cruciate and patellar.
Vessels – popliteal artery.
Nerves – common peroneal and tibial.
Tendons – quadriceps, hamstrings, gastrocnemius, sartorius, gracilis.
Menisci.

A2. a. Residual deformity.
b. Vascular status (dorsalis pedis/posterior tibial pulse). Any concern regarding the vascular status of the limb requires urgent transfer to an appropriate medical facility. Angiography might be indicated to assess for evidence of a vascular injury and its location.
c. Neurological status (common peroneal/tibial nerve).

A3. a. Knee dislocation/multi-ligament injury.
b. Posterolateral corner injury.

A4. a. Significant varus or valgus laxity in extension.
b. Significant recurvatum on extension.

A5. Advantages include:
a. Speed of obtaining imaging.
b. Possibility of identifying a tibial plateau fracture.
c. Can look for evidence of capsular injury (Segond fracture).
d. Can look for evidence of a posterolateral corner injury (fibular head fracture or avulsion).
e. Can look for evidence of other ligament avulsions (PCL/ACL/MCL).
Disadvantages include:
a. Underestimation of severity of ligament injury.
b. Failure to identify meniscal tears.

A6. In the acute situation, other serious injuries need to be excluded and the neurovascular status of the limb should be documented and monitored. Immobilisation splints should be used and transfer to the nearest appropriate medical facility arranged. Investigations should include plain x-rays and MRI. Following a thorough neurovascular assessment of the limb, the immediate priority in the dislocated knee is reduction and temporary stabilisation of the joint, using appropriate anaesthesia or sedation with external splintage. After reduction, the vascular status of the limb should be reassessed.

Injuries of this severity should be managed by surgeons with expertise in complex ligament reconstruction. In the absence of a neurovascular injury, most specialists would advocate primary repair of the capsular and collateral structures, which can be achieved by ligament reattachment, augmentation or a combination of techniques. Associated fractures of the tibial plateau or distal femur can be treated with appropriate fixation methods.

Once initial stability and limb viability has been achieved, delayed reconstruction of the cruciate ligaments can be carried out as a staged procedure, if required, once the swelling of the knee has resolved and motion has been regained.

A7. In most cases ligament reconstruction is required. Although some specialists would recommend an acute reconstruction of the cruciate ligament component injury, the degree of capsular injury must be assessed. Attempts to perform arthroscopic surgery before capsular healing increase the risk of fluid extravasation and may precipitate the development of a compartment syndrome. Reconstruction can be performed using arthroscopically assisted techniques, once the swelling around the knee has reduced and a normal range of movement returned. Various techniques and fixation methods are available, including the use of both autologous and allograft tendons.

11

The patella and patellofemoral joint

The patella is the largest of the sesamoid bones. The quadriceps tendon attaches to its upper border (base), whilst the non-extensile patellar ligament attaches to the apex.

Patellofemoral joint

This forms the anterior part of the knee articulation. It is a synovial gliding joint between the posterior surface of the patella, covered by articular cartilage and the trochlear (patellar) surface of the femur. The synovial cavity is in direct continuity with that of the femoro-tibial joint.

Movement between articular surfaces

During knee flexion and extension, the *patella remains fixed* whilst the *trochlear surface of the femur moves on the patella.* Thus, during knee flexion the *femur* moves progressively *up* the patella until finally, in full flexion, it articulates with a small vertical facet on the medial border of the patella. From the alternative perspective, the *patella* moves *down* the femur. Only 30% of the patella is in contact with the trochlear surface at any particular position (see Figures 58 and 59).

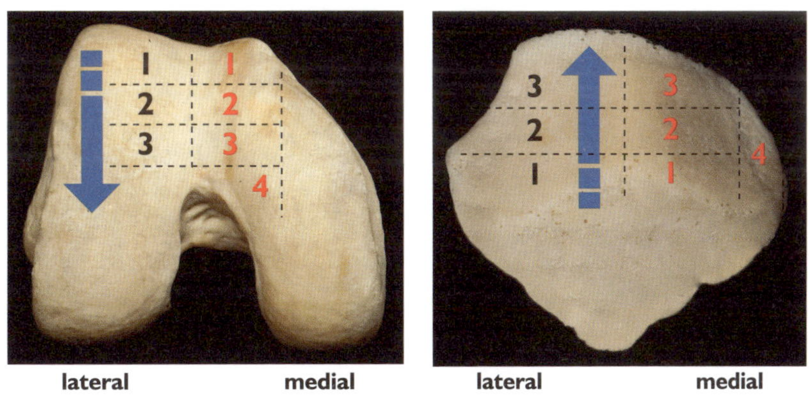

Figure 58: Articulation of the patella with the femur

Note: With the knee extended, the most anterior part of the femoral condyles (trochlea), zone 1, articulates with the most inferior part of the patella, zone 1. With completion of flexion, zone 4 on the femur is in contact with zone 4 on the medial side of the patella (see Figure 58).

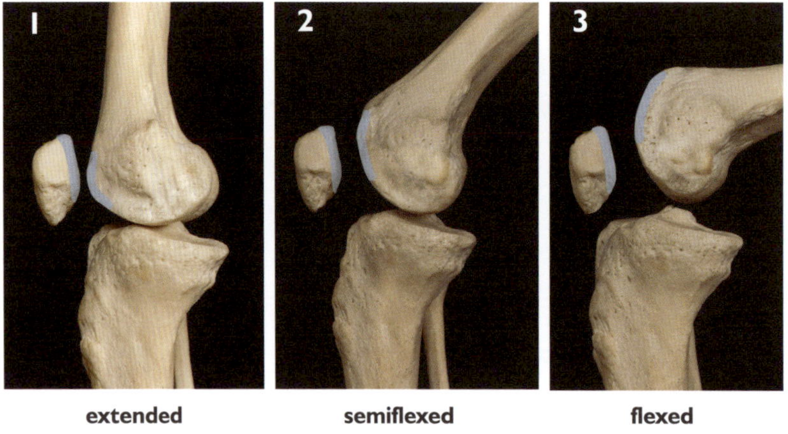

Figure 59: Movement of the trochlea of the femur in relation to the patella

Q-angle

The patella, which is an asymmetrical wedge shape, lies in the reciprocally shaped trochlea on the front of the femur. When the knee joint is extended the pull of the quadriceps tendon on the upper border of the patella tends to cause it to be displaced laterally. This is the result of angulation of the femur, whose long axis lies obliquely as compared with the long axis of the tibia and fibula, which is vertical. The angulation of the femur is due to the head articulating proximally with the acetabulum of the pelvis. Since the pelvis is wider in the female, the angulation of the femur is greater in the female. The angulation has been quantified as the 'Q angle'.

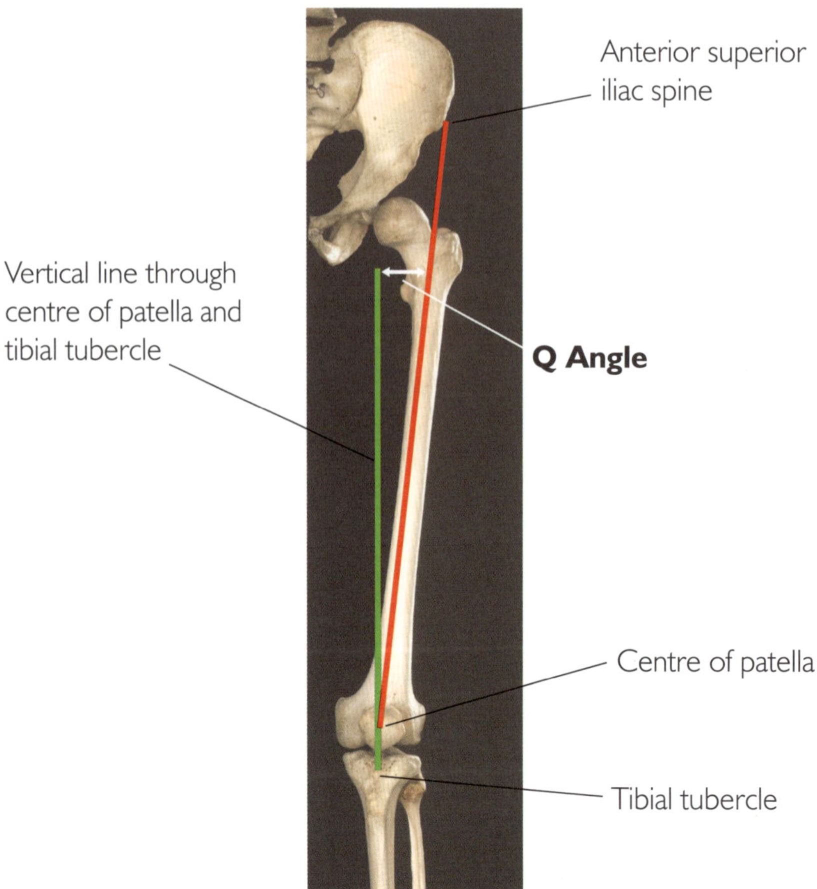

Figure 60: Calculation of the Q-angle

The angulation of the femur is measured as the 'Q angle'. It is usually less than 10° in males but up to 15° in females (see Figure 60). Higher Q angle has been proposed as a potential risk factor for patellofemoral dysfunction and injury but the clinical relevance of the Q angle has not been established.

The Q-angle is affected by several factors, including:

- Width of the pelvis
- Internal femoral rotation (anteversion)
- Genu valgum.

Factors stabilising the patella and preventing lateral displacement

1. Bony

The lateral part of the trochlear surface of the femur is more prominent and has a larger surface area compared with the medial part of the trochlea (see Figures 2a, page 6, 6c, page 15 and 62, page 84), thus preventing lateral movement. Trochlear dysplasia may lead to incongruity of the articular surfaces (see Figure 61, page 84) and consequent instability, such as a shallow trochlear groove with a flat patella or a narrow trochlear groove with a large deep patella.

2. Muscular

As compared with the vastus lateralis muscle, the vastus medialis has a larger attachment to the patella, extending along the base and down the medial border (see Figure 62, page 84), pulling it medially.

3. Ligaments

The medial and lateral patellar retinacula provide strong anchorage, the medial being particularly strong. They assist in keeping the patella firmly engaged in the trochlear groove of the femur and are formed by strong bands of the investing layer of deep fascia (see Figure 63, page 84), which fuse with the fascia covering the respective vasti muscles on each side of the knee.

In addition, the investing fascia forms thick bands that pass across the front of the patellar ligament (see Figure 63) as it descends to the tibial tuberosity. These may assist the mechanical efficiency of the ligament by preventing bow-stringing.

The space between the medial border of the patella and the medial femoral and tibial condyles has received special attention and has been described as the *medial compartment of the knee* (*Wheeless' Textbook of Orthopaedics*) and contains a ligamentous complex (Dirim et *al.* 2008) whose components are particularly important in preventing lateral patellar displacement.

The compartment is described as having three layers (Standring 2008). This concept was first described by Warren and Marshall (1979), who noted that ligaments on the medial side of the knee are condensations within tissue planes and not discrete structures. Three distinct layers are restricted to a small area, where the fascia and superficial medial ligament directly overlie the deep medial ligament. The deepest layer is formed by the capsule and deep part of the tibial collateral ligament. An intermediate layer includes the superficial part of the collateral ligament, the medial patellar retinaculum and the medial patellofemoral ligament. The outermost layer is fascia covering the sartorius muscle. The retinaculum is well defined and bilaminar (Starok et *al.* 1997).

The medial patellofemoral ligament is described as passing downwards from the medial epicondyle to the medial border of the patella and to be important in resisting lateral displacement of the patella. However it is very variable and can be a well-developed ligament or a 'mere wisp' (Warren & Marshall 1979). It has also been described as a component of the retinaculum (Starok et *al*. 1997) to merge with the tibial collateral ligament (Dirim et *al*. 2008), and as a condensation of the capsule (*Wheeless' Textbook of Orthopaedics*). Whilst three layers are described, they are not readily separated. Thus, in lateral dislocation of the patella, it is likely that damage will not be confined to just one layer and that surgical repair will involve all three layers.

Figure 61: Bilateral skyline X-ray view of left and right patella showing asymmetry.
The red arrows point to the sloping profiles of the lateral part of the trochlear surfaces. The right side is steep and is normal, whereas on the left side it is much flatter, which predisposes to instability.

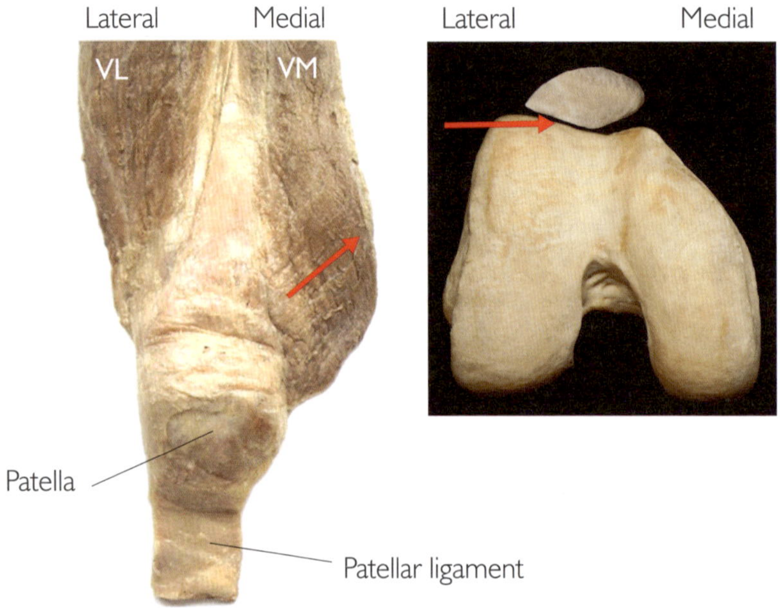

Figure 62: Muscular and bony mechanisms resisting lateral displacement of the patella

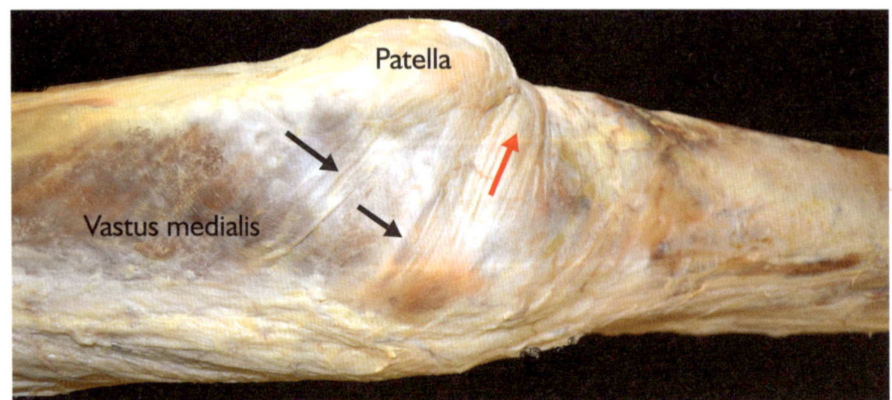

Figure 63: Medial side of the knee. The black arrows indicate fibres of the medial retinaculum and the red arrow fibres of the investing deep fascia passing across the patellar ligament.

Ossification

Ossification commences between three and six years of age. There may be only one centre of ossification but initially there are often several that coalesce into one centre. About the age of puberty, ossification is complete. It is important to note that occasionally separate centres persist (see Figure 64), especially near the supero-lateral edge of the patella, which do not fuse. These 'bipartite' or 'tripartite' patellae can easily be mistaken for a fractured patella. They are more common in males.

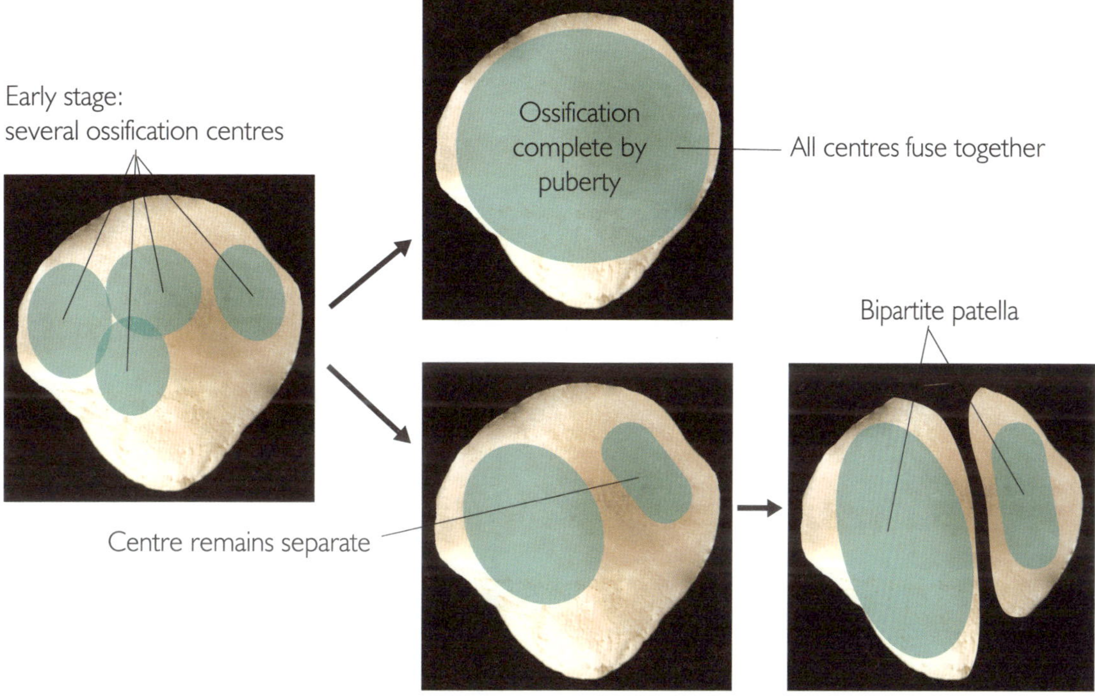

Figure 64: Ossification of the patella with formation of bipartite patella

Instability and maltracking of the patella

There are varying degrees of instability and lateral displacement of the patella during patellar movement (see Figure 65, page 86). This movement has been termed 'lateral tracking' and it often results in damage to the articulating surfaces of the patella and adjacent trochlea of the femur.

- Lateral tracking may cause damage at the lateral border (angle) of the patella, including the under surface, and to the subjacent part of the trochlear surface of the femur. With further lateral tracking, the space between the medial part of the patella and femur widens and the medial border of the patella displaces forwards (see Figure 66, page 86).
- Lateral tilting of the patella with some subluxation
- Severe subluxation
- Dislocation.

In any of these situations, there may be osteochondral damage to the trochlea and the patella. In severe dislocation, there may be fracture of the trochlea with tearing of the joint capsule and exposure of the joint cavity. The sequence of events and consequences of lateral tracking can be readily defined using MRI and examples are shown in Figures 67a, 67b and 67c.

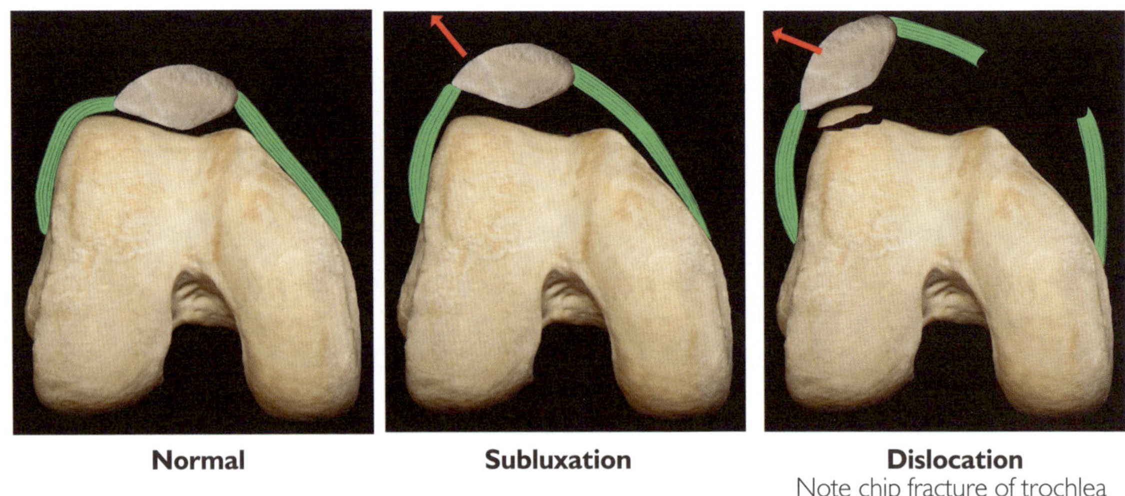

Figure 65: Types of patellar instability

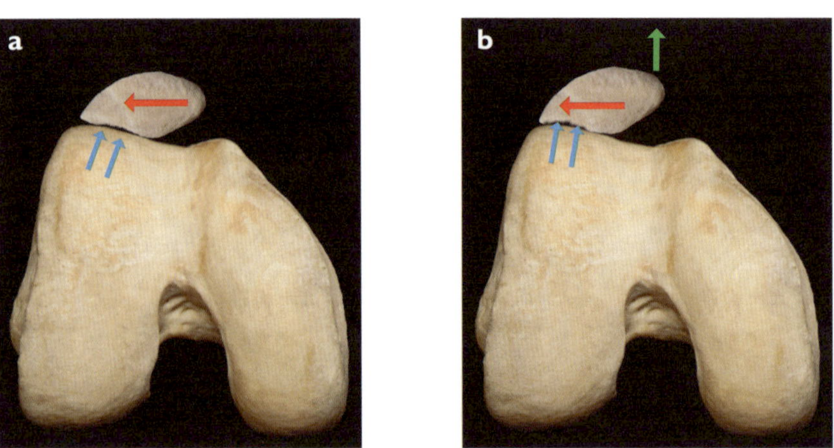

Figure 66: Pattern of patella maltracking.
As the patella moves laterally (red arrows), it impinges against the trochlea causing local damage (blue arrows). Also the medial border of the patella tilts forwards (green arrow)

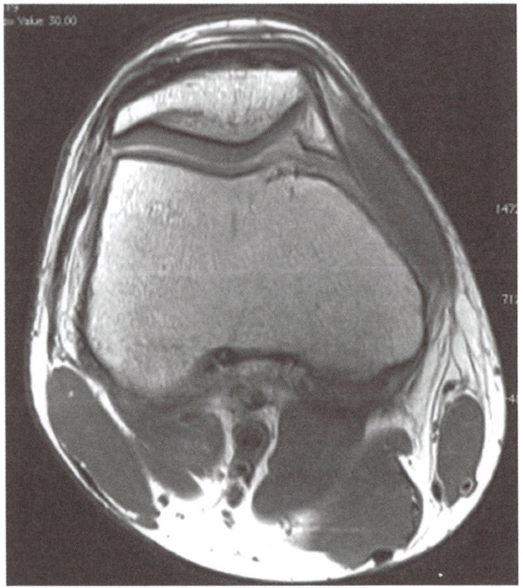

Figure 67a: Normal patella alignment on the trochlea

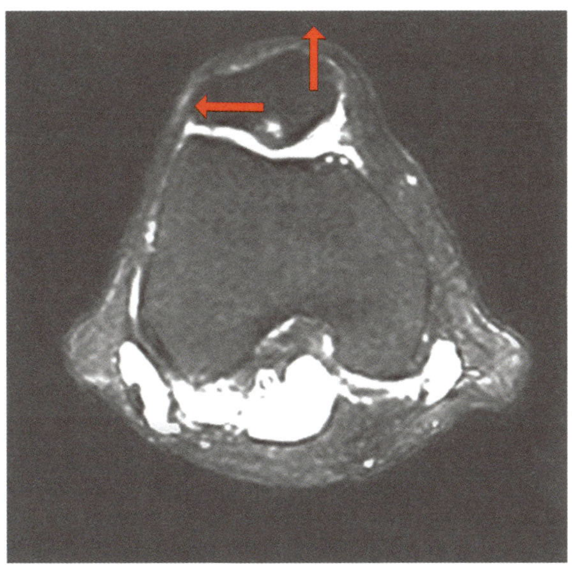

Figure 67b: MRI of a laterally positioned and tilted patella.
Compare with Figure 66. Note the subchondral bone oedema in the patella on the STIR scan.

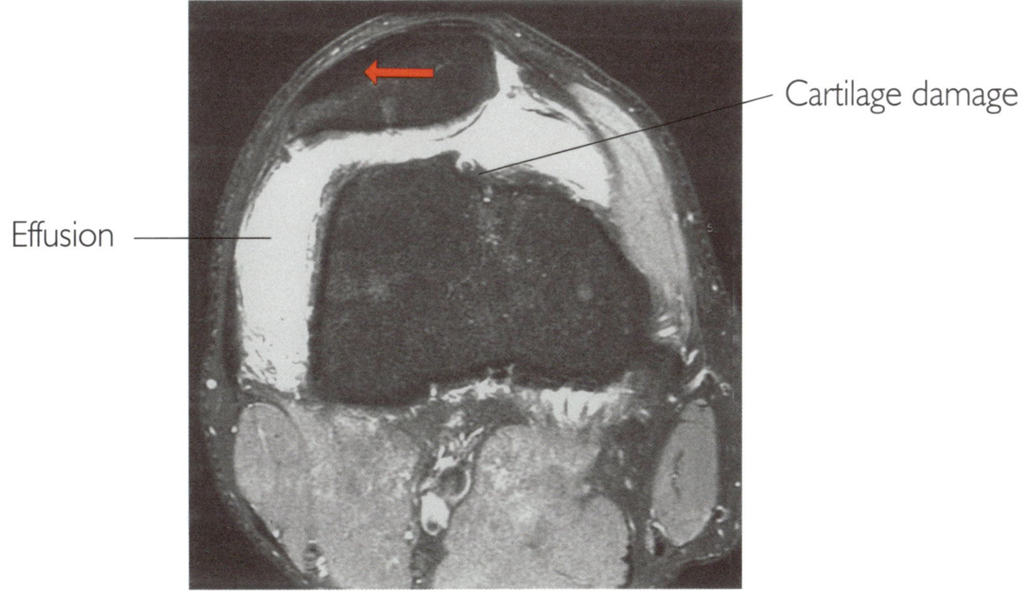

Figure 67c: T2 MRI of a laterally positioned (subluxed) patella.
Note the irregularity of the trochlea articular cartilage and the large joint effusion (white).

Problem 13

Sport – Volleyball

Clinical history

A 16-year-old girl was playing volleyball at school when she landed awkwardly from a jump, with her left knee collapsing inwards. She 'felt something move' in her knee. She was in significant pain and could see an unnatural large 'lump' on the antero-lateral side of her knee. She tried to straighten her knee but was initially unable to do so. After a short period she was able to do so and felt a clunk. Her pain, although severe, improved and the lump disappeared. The girl comes to see you three weeks later, when the knee is less painful. She is worried it 'may go again'. The patient is taking Sports Studies at school and is considering a career as a Physical Education teacher.

Q1. What is the most likely diagnosis?

Examination

There is still a small effusion in the knee.

Q2. What other key features should be assessed when examining the knee?

Investigations

Q3. Which investigations might be helpful?

Treatment

Q4. What treatment options are available?

Problem 13: Answers

Diagnosis: Patellofemoral instability

A1. Patellar dislocation

A2. a. Patellar height.

b. Patellar mobility and apprehension with lateral glide.

c. Q angle.

d. Dynamic control on squatting, especially degree of knee valgus and hip internal rotation.

e. General joint hypermobility, e.g. a Beighton's scale assessment.

A3. a. Plain x-ray, including skyline views (see Figure 61, page 84), in order to rule out large osteochondral fractures and make some assessment of trochlear and patellar morphology.

b. Long leg views – to assess alignment and varus/valgus angle at the knee.

c. An MRI scan to allow assessment of the articular surfaces (see Figures 67a, 67b and 67c), to measure the tibial tubercle/trochlear distance and to assess any damage to the medial patellofemoral ligament (MPFL).

A4. a. A conservative approach should include restoration of range of movement, restoration of quadriceps strength and control, squat, single leg squat, jump and landing exercise rehabilitation aimed at optimising pelvic, hip, knee and leg alignment and control.

b. Surgery to correct alignment abnormalities and soft tissue damage (e.g. to the MPFL) should be reserved in case of failure of conservative treatment. In more extreme cases extensor realignment surgery, or surgery to alter the trochlear morphology, may be required.

Rupture of the extensor mechanism

The extensor mechanism includes the quadriceps extensor tendon, the patella to which it attaches and the inextensible patellar ligament passing to the tibial tubercle. Working distally, there are four types of injury (Figure 68):

a. Rupture of the quadriceps tendon where it attaches to the upper border of the patella
b. A transverse fracture through the body of the patella
c. Rupture of the proximal end of the patellar ligament, together with an attached small piece of adjacent patella
d. Rupture of the distal end of the patellar ligament, or detachment of the tibial tubercle.

A similar result may occur from separation of the epiphysis due to excessive traction on the epiphysis by the lower end of the patellar ligament (see Figure 69).

Ruptures in the more proximal part of the extensor system are more common in the older population, whereas they tend to occur in the lower part in younger people.

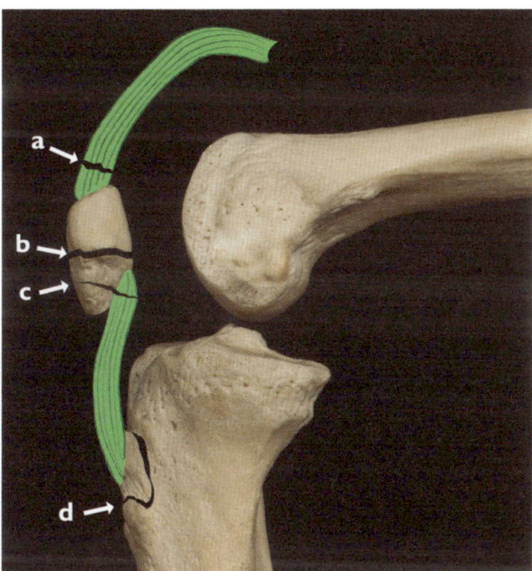

Figure 68: Sites of disruption of the knee extensor mechanism

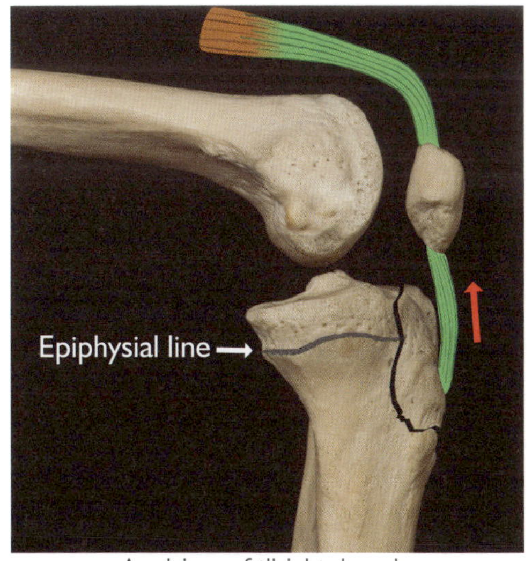

Avulsion of tibial tubercle with adjacent tibial epiphysis

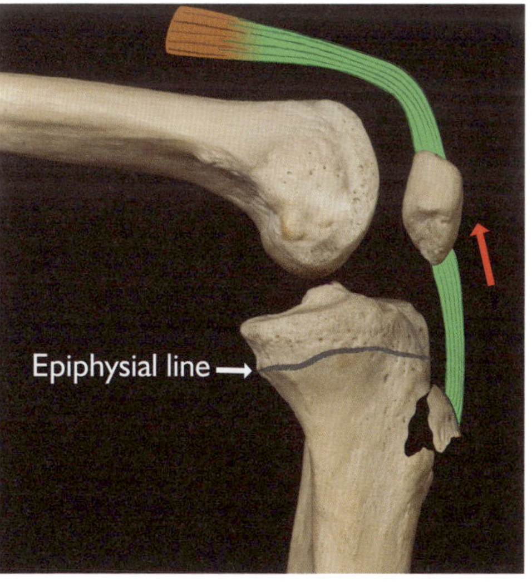

Separation of epiphysis of tibial tubercle

Figure 69: Separation of epiphyses associated with the patellar tendon

Patellar fractures

Patellar fractures can be categorised as follows:

- Transverse fracture of the body or lower pole, with separation of fragments and rupture of quadriceps tendon.
- Transverse fracture of the body or lower pole without separation of fragments and quadriceps tendon intact (see Figure 70). This is caused by direct trauma or leverage associated with violent muscular contraction of quadriceps with the knee partially flexed.
- Comminuted and chip fractures due to direct trauma.

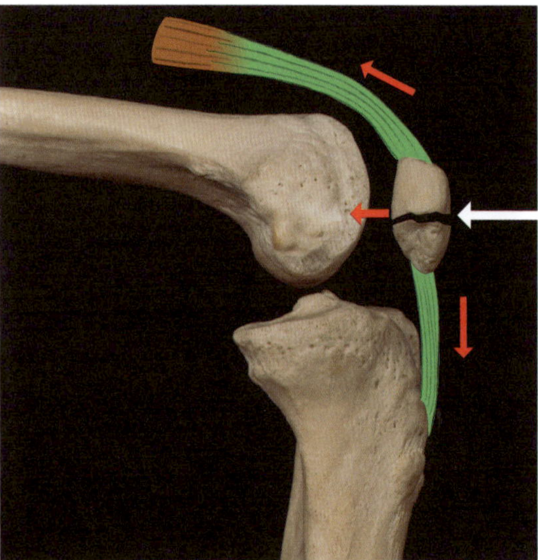

Figure 70: Transverse patella fracture

Innervation in relation to knee pain

There are two components to knee innervation: an *external* comprising the principal nerves of the region that give branches to the joint; and an *internal* comprising innervation of the various components of the joint.

The principal external innervation is from three nerves:

1. Femoral nerve (L2, 3, 4): Through branches to the quadriceps femoris, including the three vasti and the rectus femoris. These supply structures in the anterior part of the joint, including capsule, quadriceps tendon, retinacula, patella, patellar ligament, infrapatellar fat pad and plica. Injury and damage to these structures causes anterior knee pain ('runner's knee').

2. Obturator nerve (L2, 3, 4): A branch from the posterior division supplies the adductor magnus and continues to the posteromedial side of the joint. Branches supply the oblique popliteal ligament and medial side of the joint, including medial collateral ligament and medial meniscus. Damage to these structures causes medial knee pain. Since the obturator nerve also supplies the hip joint, pain may be referred from the knee to the hip (or vice versa).

3. Sciatic nerve (L4, 5, S1, 2, 3): Each of the sciatic nerve's two main terminal branches supply the knee. From the tibial nerve, genicular branches pass to the posteromedial part of the joint. They supply structures on the posterior aspect of the joint, including hamstring tendons, posterior capsule, anterior and posterior cruciate ligaments, popliteus and plantaris, damage to which causes posterior knee pain. From the common peroneal nerve, branches pass to the posterolateral side and innervate structures on the lateral side of the joint, including the lateral collateral ligament, lateral meniscus and iliotibial band. Damage to these structures causes lateral knee pain.

The critical factor in internal innervation is what types of nerve endings are found in the joint and their distribution in the various components. Essentially there are two types of ending: encapsulated, which are proprioceptive (mechanoreceptors); and free endings, which mediate pain. Damage to the former can contribute to joint instability. The distribution of these two types of endings in the joint is as follows:

- Articular cartilage – no innervation
- Subchondral bone – pain receptors
- Patella – pain endings in subchondral plate
- Capsule – pain receptors and mechanoreceptors
- Medial and lateral retinaculum – pain receptors
- Ligaments and iliotibial tract – pain receptors and mechanoreceptors
- Fat pads – pain receptors and mechanoreceptors
- Synovial membrane – pain receptors, including those that form part of the perivascular plexuses supplying blood vessels
- Meniscus – no receptors in the fibro-cartilaginous medial thin part of the meniscus. Pain receptors in the thicker peripheral vascularised part adjacent to the capsule; also some mechanoreceptors.

This summary is based on a number of reports, including Biedert *et al.* (1992), Hirasawa *et al.* (2000), Mine *et al.* (2000), Witonski *et al.* (2005), Wojtys *et al.* (1990), Biedert & Sanchis-Alfonso (2002).
Thus, apart from the articular cartilage itself, injury to virtually all the knee structures commonly involved in sports injuries generates pain as a consequence of their intrinsic innervation.

12

Fracture patterns of proximal tibia and knee epiphyses

Fractures of the tibia involving the knee joint

Indirect trauma resulting in excessive forces acting at the proximal end of the tibia can produce a variety of fractures, some of which involve the knee joint itself. The mechanism is shown in Figure 71. They may be simple, comminuted or depressed and examples are shown in Figures 72 and 73. In some injuries residual arthritic changes may result, due to chondral and subchondral injury.

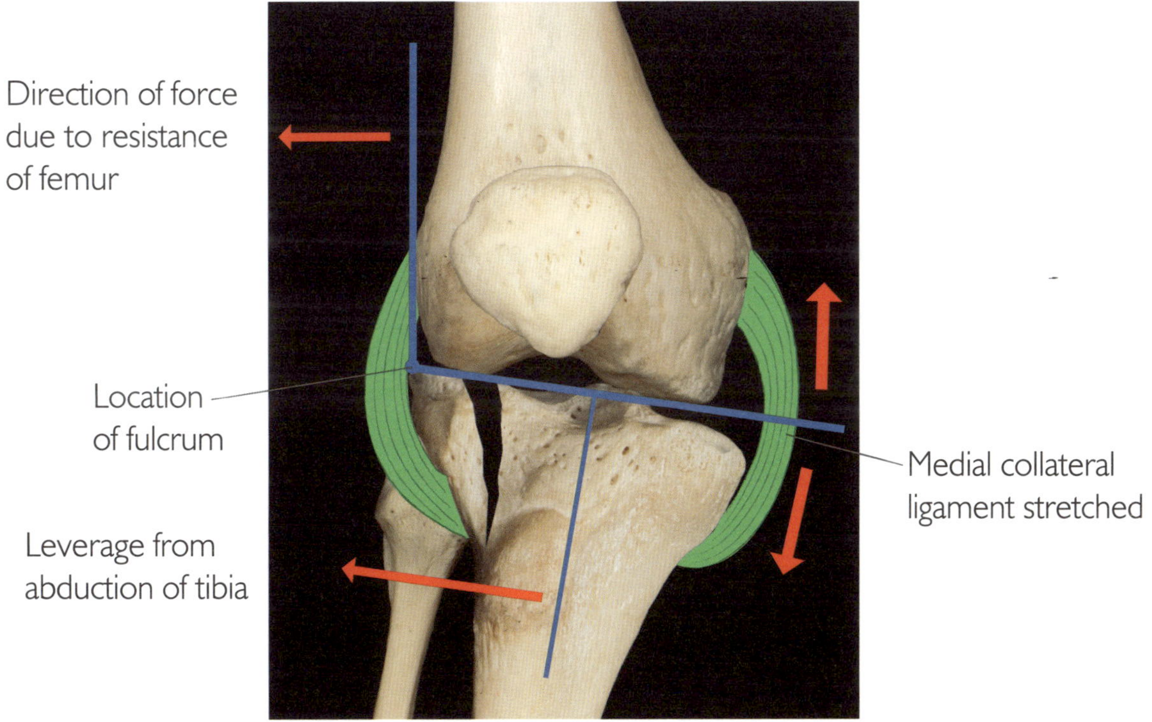

Figure 71: Mechanism of proximal-lateral tibial abduction fracture

Note: In adduction fractures, a mirror image of the forces and injuries shown in the diagram applies.

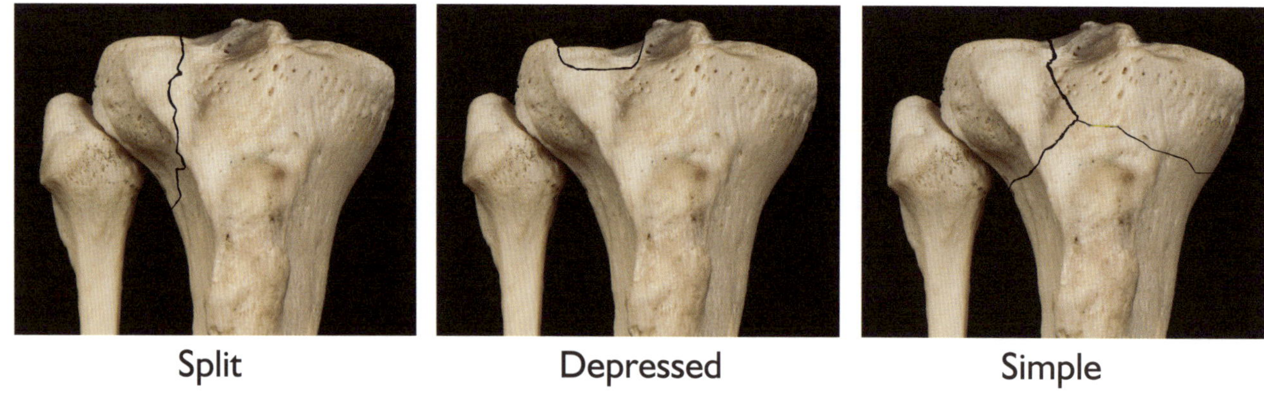

Figure 72: Examples of fracture patterns in the proximal tibia and tibial plateau

Problem 14

Sport – Basketball

Clinical history

A 25-year-old female basketball player collides awkwardly with another player, landing on her left leg with her opponent's weight on top of her. The knee is seen to buckle into valgus. She screams out in pain and is unable to weight bear. Within a short period, her knee is significantly swollen.

Q1. What is the most likely diagnosis?

Examination

The leg is swollen and any attempt to straighten it results in significant pain. The player is complaining of some numbness in her foot.

Q2. What is the appropriate initial treatment?

Q3. What neurovascular structures must you assess?

Investigations

The player is transferred to the emergency department.

Q4. Which investigations might be appropriate?

Treatment

Investigation reveals a tibial plateau fracture.

Q5. What treatment options are available?

Q6. What is the prognosis following this injury?

Problem 14: Answers

Diagnosis: Tibial plateau fracture

A1. a. Tibial plateau fracture. These usually occur as a result of high-energy varus or valgus forces on the knee. They often occur in conjunction with cruciate or collateral ligament injuries. These injuries can occur in the elderly as low-energy osteoporotic fractures.

b. Knee dislocation.
c. Patellar dislocation.

A2. a. POLICE regimen.
b. Splinting.
c. Early transfer to a medical facility.
d. Pain relief.

A3. a. Common peroneal nerve.
a. Dorsalis pedis artery pulse in the foot and posterior tibial artery pulse at the ankle in case of damage to the popliteal artery.

A4. a. An x-ray. A lateral view will often show a fat/fluid level in case of a fracture. A tibial plateau fracture is usually visible on the AP view.
b. An MRI scan (see Figure 73). Occult fractures can occur and not be visible on a standard radiograph. The MRI can also reveal associated injuries to ligaments and menisci.

A5. a. If there is minimal displacement of the fracture fragments, treatment using a cast or splint, with a period of restricted weight-bearing, may be possible.
b. In fractures with significant displacement, surgery may be required to realign the joint surface.

A6. The prognosis will depend on the energy involved, on the complexity of the fracture, the degree of damage to the chondral surfaces and any associated meniscal injury. Even with optimal treatment, it is probable that the knee will develop early degenerative change in the affected compartment.

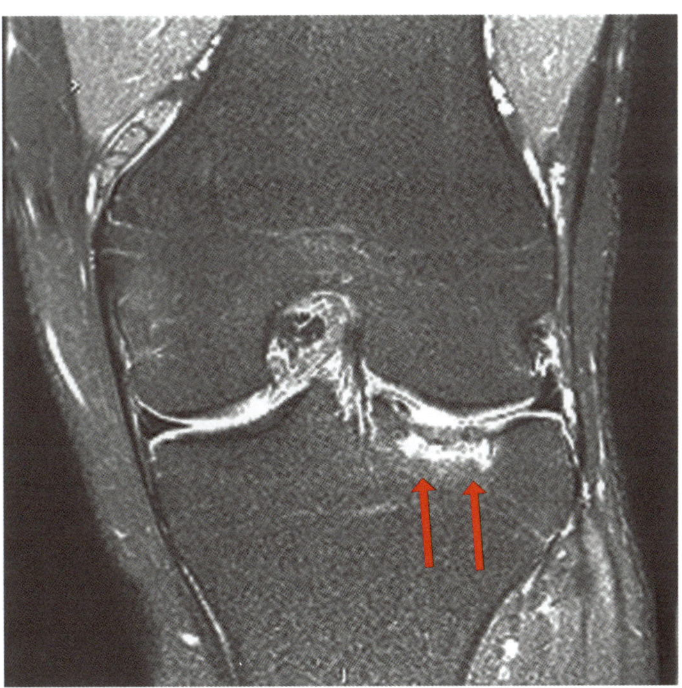

Figure 73: MRI confirming lateral tibial plateau impaction fracture (red arrows)

Location and fusion times of knee epiphyses

To avoid the pitfalls in interpreting x-radiographs and scans of knee injuries in the young sport enthusiast, it is important to be aware of the location and appearance of epiphyses in the region of the knee and when fusion occurs with the main shaft of the bone (see Figures 74 and 75).

Femur

A single epiphysis for the femoral condyles and trochlea fuses with the shaft between 18 and 20 years of age.

Tibia

A separate secondary centre for ossification in the tibial tubercle often appears about the twelfth year and usually fuses with the main epiphysis for the tibial condyles during the sixteenth to eighteenth years. Finally, the main epiphysis at the upper end of the tibia fuses with the shaft during the sixteenth to eighteenth years. Note: Patella ossification is considered previously on page 85.

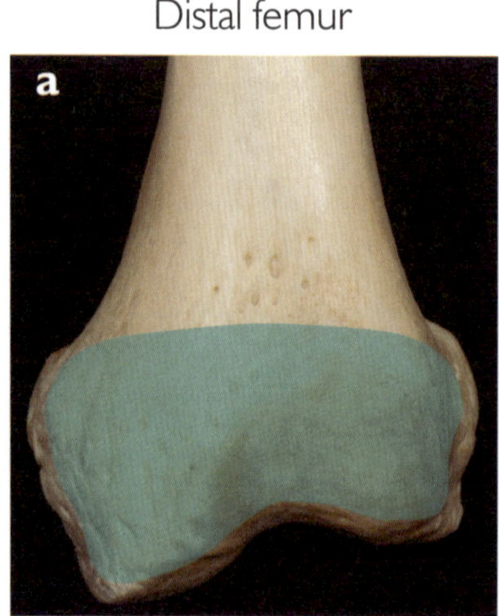

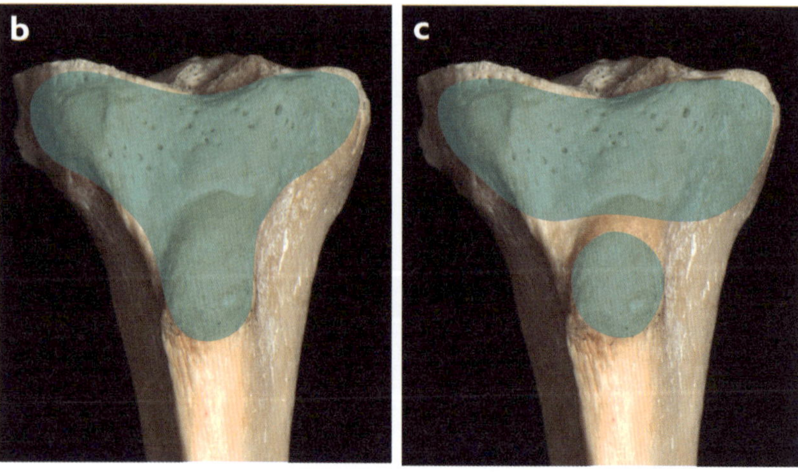

Figure 74: Location and fusion times of knee epiphyses.

Note: Tibial epiphysis may take one of two forms (b or c). Compare a, b and c with x-ray appearance in Figure 75.

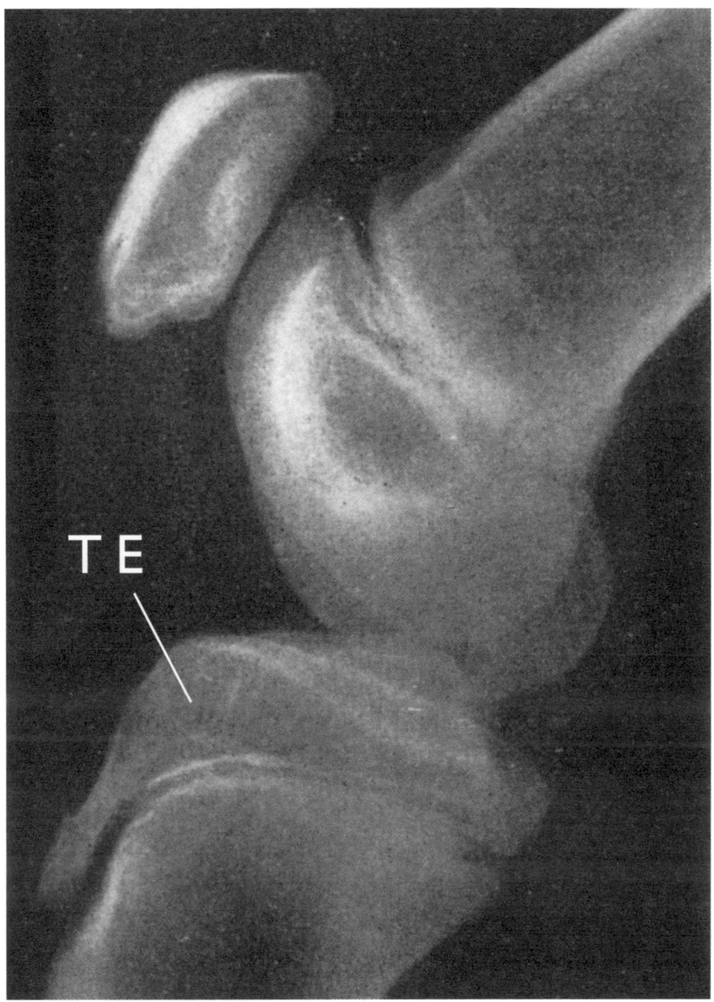

Figure 75: Lateral radiograph of lower femoral and upper tibial epiphysis (TE) in a 12-year-old boy. Note: It includes the centre for the tibial tubercle. There is a single epiphysis at the lower end of the femur.

References

Arnoczky, S.P. & Warren, R.F. (1982). Microvasculature of the human meniscus. *American Journal of Sports Medicine.* **10**, 90–95.

Biedert, R.M. & Sanchis-Alfonso, V. (2002). Sources of anterior knee pain. *Clinical Sports Medicine.* **21**, 335–47, vii.

Biedert, R.M., Stauffer, E. & Friederich, N.F. (1992). Occurrence of free nerve endings in the soft tissue of the knee joint. A histologic investigation. *American Journal of Sports Medicine.* **20**, 430–33.

Bout-Tabaku, S. & Best, T.M. (2010). The adolescent knee and risk for osteoarthritis – an opportunity or responsibility for sport medicine physicians? *Current Sports Medicine Reports.* **9**, 329–31.

Cook, J.L. & Purdam, C.R. (2008). Is tendon pathology a continuum? A pathology model to explain the clinical presentation of load-induced tendinopathy. *British Journal of Sports Medicine.* **43**, 409–16.

Dirim, B., Haghighi, P., Trudell, D., Portes, G. & Resnick, D. (2008). Medial patellofemoral ligament: cadaveric investigation of anatomy with MRI, MR arthrography, and histologic correlation. *American Journal of Radiology.* **191**, 490–98.

Eckstein, F., Hudelmaier, M. & Putz, R. (2006). The effects of exercise on human articular cartilage. *Journal of Anatomy.* **208**, 491–512.

Fairclough, J., Hayashi, K., Toumi, H., Lyons, K., Bydder, G., Phillips, N., Best, T.M. & Benjamin, M. (2006). The functional anatomy of the iliotibial band during flexion and extension of the knee: implications for understanding iliotibial band syndrome. *Journal of Anatomy.* **208**, 309–16.

Fairclough, J., Hayashi, K., Toumi, H., Lyons, K., Bydder, G., Phillips, N., Best, T.M. & Benjamin, M. (2007). Is iliotibial band syndrome really a friction syndrome? *Journal of Science and Medicine in Sport.* **10**, 74–6; discussion 77–8.

Ferber, R., Noehren, B., Hamill, J. & Davis, I.S. (2010). Competitive female runners with a history of iliotibial band syndrome demonstrate atypical hip and knee kinematics. *Journal of Orthopaedic Sports Physical Therapy.* **40**, 52–8.

Garcia-Valtuille, R., Abascal, F., Cerezal, L., Garcia-Valtuille, A., Pereda, T., Canga, A. & Cruz, A. (2002). Anatomy and MR imaging appearances of synovial plicae of the knee. *Radiographics: a review publication of the Radiological Society of North America, Inc.* **22**, 775–84.

Getgood, A. & Robertson, A. (2010). Meniscal tears, repairs and replacement: A current concepts review. *Orthopaedics and Trauma.* **24**, 121–28.

Harris, P.F. & Ranson, C.A. (2008). *Atlas of Living and Surface Anatomy for Sports Medicine.* Edinburgh: Churchill Livingstone.

Hirasawa, Y., Okajima, S., Ohta, M. & Tokioka, T. (2000). Nerve distribution to the human knee joint: anatomical and immunohistochemical study. *International Orthopedics.* **24**, 1–4.

Horky, D. (1981). Submicroscopic structure of the human synovial membrane. *Acta Veterinaria Brno.* **50**, 3–25.

Levick, J.R. & McDonald, J.N. (1995). Fluid movement across synovium in healthy joints: role of synovial fluid macromolecules. *Annals of Rheumatic Disease.* **54**, 417–23.

Lobenhoffer, P., Biedert, R., Stauffer, E., Lattermann C., Gerlich, T.G. & Muller, W. (1996). Occurrence and distribution of free nerve endings in the distal iliotibial tract system of the knee. *Knee Surgery, Sports Traumatology, Arthroscopy.* **4**, 111–15.

Mine, T., Kimura, M., Sakka, A. & Kawai, S. (2000). Innervation of nociceptors in the menisci of the knee joint: an immunohistochemical study. *Archives of Orthopaedic and Trauma Surgery.* **120**, 201–4.

Perera, J.R., Gikas, P.D. & Bentley, G. (2012). The present state of treatments for articular cartilage defects in the knee. *Annals of the Royal College of Surgery of England.* **94**, 381–87.

Radhakrishna, M., Macdonald, P., Davidson, M., Hodgekinson, R. & Craton, N. (2004). Isolated popliteus injury in a professional football player. *Clinical Journal of Sport Medicine: Official Journal of the Canadian Academy of Sport Medicine.* **14**, 365–67.

Robertson, A., Nutton, R.W. & Keating, J.F. (2006). Dislocation of the knee. *The Journal of Bone and Joint Surgery (British Volume).* **88**, 706–11.

Standring, S. (2008). Ed. *Gray's Anatomy.* 40th Edn. Edinburgh: Churchill Livingstone, Chapter 82, Knee pp. 1399–1400.

Starok, M., Lenchik, L., Trudell, D. & Resnick, D. (1997). Normal patellar retinaculum: MR and Sonographic imaging with cadaver correlation. *American Journal of Radiology.* **168**, 1493–9.

Toumi, H., Higashiyama, I., Suzuki, D., Kumai, T., Bydder, G., McGonagle, D., Emery, P., Fairclough, J. & Benjamin, M. (2006). Regional variations in human patellar trabecular architecture and the structure of the proximal patellar tendon enthesis. *Journal of Anatomy*. **208**, 47–57.

Warren, L.F. & Marshall, J.L. (1979). The supporting structures and layers on the medial side of the knee: an anatomical analysis. *Journal of Bone and Joint Surgery*. **61A**, 56–62.

Wheeless' Textbook of Orthopaedics. Medial patellofemoral ligament. www.wheelessonline.com

Witonski, D., Wagrowska-Danilewicz, M. & Raczynska-Witonska, G. (2005). Distribution of substance P nerve fibers in osteoarthritis knee joint. *Polish Journal of Pathology*. **56**, 203–6

Wojtys, E.M., Beaman, D.N., Glover, R.A. & Janda, D. (1990). Innervation of the human knee joint by substance-P fibers. *Arthroscopy*. **6**, 254–63.

Index